MANUAL OF **PLEURAL PROCEDURES**

HENRI G. COLT, M.D.
Associate Professor of Medicine,
Chief, Interventional Pulmonology,
Division of Pulmonary and Critical Medicine,
Department of Medicine, University of California
San Diego Medical Center, San Diego, California

PRAVEEN N. MATHUR, M.B.B.S.
Professor of Medicine, Department of Medicine,
Division of Pulmonary and Critical Care Medicine,
Indiana University Medical Center, Indianapolis, Indiana

LIPPINCOTT WILLIAMS & WILKINS
A **Wolters Kluwer** Company
Philadelphia • Baltimore • New York • London
Buenos Aires • Hong Kong • Sydney • Tokyo

Acquisitions Editor: Joyce-Rachel John
Developmental Editor: Keith Donnellan
Manufacturing Manager: Kevin Watt
Production Manager: Robert Pancotti
Production Editor: Melanie Bennitt
Cover Designer: Kevin Kall
Indexer: Frances Lennie
Compositor: Lippincott Williams & Wilkins Desktop Division
Printer: RR Donnelley, Crawfordsville

Printed in the United States of America

9 8 7 6 5 4 3 2 1

Library of Congress Cataloging-in-Publication Data

Manual of pleural procedures / editors, Henri G. Colt, Praveen N. Mathur.
p. cm.
Includes bibliographical references and index.
ISBN 0-7817-1476-1
1. Pleura—Diseases—Handbooks, manuals, etc. 2. Pleura—Biopsy—Handbooks, manuals, etc. I. Colt, Henri G. II. Mathur, Praveen N.
[DNLM: 1. Pleural Diseases—diagnosis. 2. Pleural Diseases—therapy. 3. Physical Examination—methods. 4. Biopsy, Needle. 5. Thoracostomy. WF 700]
RC751.M36 1999
616.2′5—dc21
DNLM/DLC
for Library of Congress 98-47494
CIP

CONTENTS

Foreword *by Deborah Shure* vii

Foreword *by Richard Light* ix

Preface xi

Acknowledgments xiii

I. Background

1 Practical Anatomy and Physiology of the Thoracic Cage and Pleura 3

2 Physical Examination of the Chest Wall, Lungs, and Pleura 13

3 Radiology of the Pleura 21

4 Ultrasonography of the Pleura 37

5 Thoracic Drainage Devices 45

6 Skin Degerming, Disinfection, and Sterilization Techniques 53

7 Pharmacologic Agents 61

8 Primer of Differential Diagnosis of Pleural Diseases . . 79

II. Pleural Procedures

9 Thoracentesis 93

10 Closed-Needle Pleural Biopsy 105

11 Fine-Needle Aspiration Biopsy 115

12 Closed-Tube Thoracostomy Using Small-Bore Chest Tubes 127

13 Closed-Tube Thoracostomy Using Large-Bore Chest Tubes 139

14 Bedside Pleurodesis 155

15 Thoracoscopy 163

Appendix: Instrument Manufacturers 179

Subject Index 181

MANUAL OF **PLEURAL PROCEDURES**

FOREWORD

A procedure manual should ideally provide sufficient background to enable the reader to understand theory, indications, and contraindications, and to provide detailed, practical information about the procedure itself. The *Manual of Pleural Procedures* meets the highest goals one can set for such a manual.

The initial chapters deal concisely but completely with anatomy, physiology, physical examination, and imaging in a way that conveys information essential to understanding the performance of the procedures described later. The imaging information is particularly helpful with a comprehensive description of newer computed tomographic (CT) and ultrasound techniques. The emphasis on the relevance of CT findings to different pleural disease processes should be particularly useful.

The clinical approach to procedures begins with general information about the differential diagnosis of pleural diseases, a helpful approach when considering appropriate diagnostic techniques. Other general chapters on disinfection, instrument sterilization, and patient anesthesia provide useful information for all the procedures detailed in later chapters.

The range of procedures covered is comprehensive, with excellent illustrations that should enable skilled persons to take on new procedures and aid trainees in understanding how to perform these essential diagnostic techniques. The manual provides important detail at every step. The "before," "during," and "after" approach used for each procedure is outstanding and ensures a thorough approach to the patient and to specimen handling, an often neglected area. The section on securing a chest tube is one of the best descriptions of the suture technique available.

Importantly, equipment is described well and comparisons among devices are clear. Distinctive black and white photographs of the equipment help to discern. The strengths and weaknesses of various devices are clearly presented, which is important in understanding possible complications.

The overall organization of the chapters is excellent for educational purposes. The sections at the end of each chapter, which list clinical pearls and answers to questions "heard on the wards," provide true hands-on clinical teaching that is refreshing and interesting. The issues raised include both critical and lighthearted ones, such as my favorite, "How do I avoid embarrassing myself during a surgical scrub?"

Although most of the procedures described in this manual have been around for many years, the organization, detail, and updated information provided is essential. With the exception of thoracoscopy, which requires considerable training, most procedures could be performed by a skilled person based on the information provided here. This work should serve as a practical and educational standard for some time to come.

Deborah Shure, M.D., F.C.C.P.
Professor of Medicine
The University of Mississippi School of Medicine
Jackson, Mississippi

FOREWORD

Physicians frequently encounter pleural problems in the practice of medicine. Pleural effusions complicate many diseases including congestive heart failure, cirrhosis, metastatic malignancy, mesothelioma, pneumonia, collagen vascular diseases, and abdominal infections. Pneumothorax occurs in patients with and without lung disease (secondary spontaneous pneumothorax and primary spontaneous pneumothorax, respectively), resulting from trauma (traumatic pneumothorax), and resulting from diagnostic or therapeutic maneuvers (iatrogenic pneumothorax). Chest tubes are used after most thoracic surgical procedures as treatment for pneumothorax and as treatment for a pleural effusion.

Drs. Henri Colt and Praveen Mathur have prepared the *Manual of Pleural Procedures* to aid physicians, nurses, and physicians' assistants caring for patients with pleural diseases. They devote the first few chapters to the anatomy and imaging of the pleural space. Subsequently, they summarize thoracic drainage procedures and the pharmacologic agents used in treating their patients. Lastly, they describe various procedures, including thoracentesis, closed-needle biopsy of the pleura, fine-needle aspiration of the lung, closed-tube thoracostomy using small- and large-bore chest tubes, pleurodesis, and thoracoscopy.

Unique aspects of this manual are the sections labeled "Clinical Pearls" and "Heard on the Wards" at the end of each chapter. The latter section poses questions frequently asked on the ward and provides articulate answers. Additionally, the summaries of the material required for each procedure are particularly useful. This is a comprehensive manual that should be invaluable to medical personnel caring for their patients with pleural problems.

Richard W. Light, M.D.
Professor of Medicine
Vanderbilt University
Nashville, Tennessee

PREFACE

The purpose of this manual is to give physicians a practical, step-by-step guide of various techniques and procedures to diagnose and treat patients with pleural disease. To achieve this goal, we divide the text into two sections. The first section gives readers essential, basic knowledge of anatomy, physiology, clinical diagnosis, equipment, and imaging methods warranted in evaluating patients with pleural processes. We devote the second section to a descriptive "How it's done" for invasive procedures such as thoracentesis, closed-needle pleural biopsy, fine-needle aspiration biopsy, small- and large-bore chest tube insertion, bedside pleurodesis, and thoracoscopy.

To facilitate ease-of-use and readability, we similarly design most chapters to address indications, contraindications, patient preparation, equipment, procedural techniques, and complications. Certain words or phrases in each chapter are presented in bold type for easy access. Bullet lists, guidelines to be used before, during, and after intervention, and management algorithms lead the reader step-by-step through each diagnostic and therapeutic intervention. Within this framework we delineate current modalities, yet occasionally, we challenge conventional teachings, such as "stepping" over the rib during thoracentesis.

Because we identify more readily with true-life images than with schematic reproductions, we frequently provide black and white photographs of patients, equipment, and techniques instead of line drawings. We hope the reader will agree that a picture is often worth a thousand words. Many figures are unique in their genre, especially for a manual this size.

In addition, we list a handful of clinically relevant comments toward the end of each chapter. A collection of questions that we have "heard on the wards" follows these "clinical pearls," accompanied by short, cut-to-the-chase answers identical to those we provide to students, house officers, and colleagues every day. A brief, annotated selection of articles for recommended reading is easily found at the end of each chapter. This bibliography humbly intends to encourage physicians, nurses, technicians, and students to plunge even more deeply into the fascinating, often misunderstood world of pleural procedures.

ACKNOWLEDGMENTS

Sincere thanks to my parents and to my wife Edwige, whose wisdom I admire, and to our editor Joyce-Rachel John, who unhesitatingly shared our vision for this manual. My most sincere gratitude also goes to Anne Powers, N.P., who has become the anchor of my Interventional Pulmonology service at UCSD Medical Center.

Henri G. Colt

I give thanks to Ms. Cherry Smith of the endoscopy suites at Indiana University Hospital for her patience and help in developing various new techniques. Also, with immense gratitude I recall the patience and understanding of my wife Pratima and my children Anu and Anita. Without their encouragement this project would not have been completed.

Praveen N. Mathur

I. BACKGROUND

1. PRACTICAL ANATOMY AND PHYSIOLOGY OF THE THORACIC CAGE AND PLEURA

Anatomy of the Thoracic Cage

The thoracic cage is made up of 12 pairs of ribs, 10 pairs of costal cartilage, 12 thoracic vertebrae, and the sternum. The 11 intercostal spaces are wider anteriorly than posteriorly. Each intercostal space contains vessels, nerves, and muscles. Along the anterolateral chest, the 10th rib can usually be felt most inferiorly in a thin person. More posteriorly, the 11th and 12th floating ribs may be palpable.

The thoracic cage is separated from the neck by the superior thoracic aperture, through which pass the great vessels, the esophagus, and the trachea. It is separated from the abdomen by the diaphragm, which forms the inferior limit of the thoracic cage. The **angle of Louis**, noted at the junction between the manubrium and body of the sternum, lies at the level of the second rib. The space just below this rib is the 2nd intercostal space.

The dome-shaped **diaphragm** is actually made up of two muscles connected medially by a fibrous septum. A peripheral muscular portion is wrapped around a central tendon. The superior aspect of this tendon is partially fused with the fibrous pericardium. During inspiration, the diaphragm contracts, pulling the central tendon downward to increase the vertical diameter of the thorax. The peripheral portion of the diaphragm arises from the margins of the thoracic outlet formed by the costal margins, the body of the 12th thoracic vertebra, and the xiphisternal joint.

The peripheral aspect of each hemidiaphragm and the parietal pleura are innervated by intercostal nerves, whereas the central portion of each hemidiaphragm is innervated by a **phrenic nerve**. The dome of each hemidiaphragm rests at approximately the 5th intercostal space anteriorly and at the 8th intercostal space posteriorly in the erect position. Because the hemidiaphragms usually function as a unit, they move inferiorly up to 2 cm during contraction, increasing the vertical dimension of the thoracic cage during inspiration. The curvature of the diaphragm forms a narrow recess at its periphery into which the lung does not extend. This is called the **costodiaphragmatic recess**. Medially, a similar recess is formed anterior to the heart. This is called the **costomediastinal recess**. These recesses are often referred to as the costophrenic and cardiophrenic angles.

The **major muscles of the anterolateral chest** are the intercostal muscles, but also the pectoralis major muscle (which arises from the medial half of the clavicle, the costal margin of the sternum, and the 2nd to 6th ribs, extending to the greater tubercle of the humerus), the serratus anterior muscle (whose muscular digitations extend from the upper eight ribs to the vertebral border of the scapula), and the pectoralis minor muscle (arising from 2nd to 6th ribs and inserting onto the coracoid process of the scapula) (Fig. 1-1).

The **major muscles of the posterolateral chest** are the trapezius muscle (which originates on the occipital bone and spines of the C7 T12 vertebrae to insert on the clavicle, acromion, and spine of the scapula), the latissimus dorsi muscle (which extends from the iliac crest and lower six thoracic vertebrae to insert into the bicipital groove of the humerus), the rhomboideus major and minor muscles (arising from the C7 T5 vertebrae and extending to the vertebral border of the scapula), and the serratus anterior and posterior muscles (Fig. 1-2).

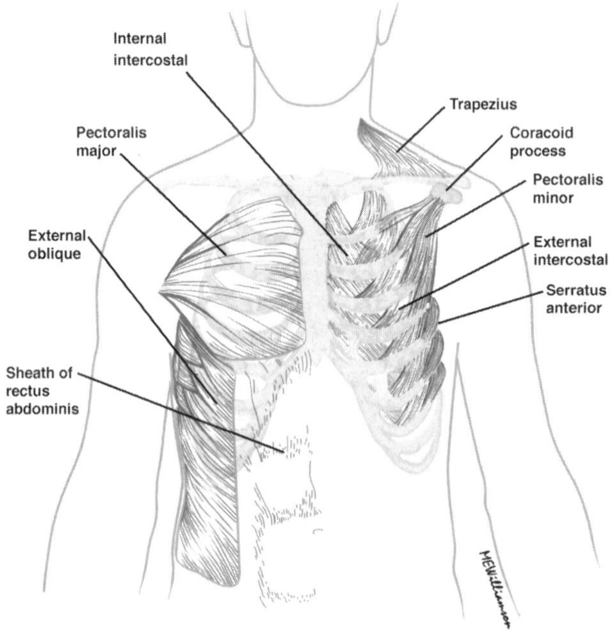

FIG. 1-1. Anterior chest wall anatomy and major muscles of inspiration.

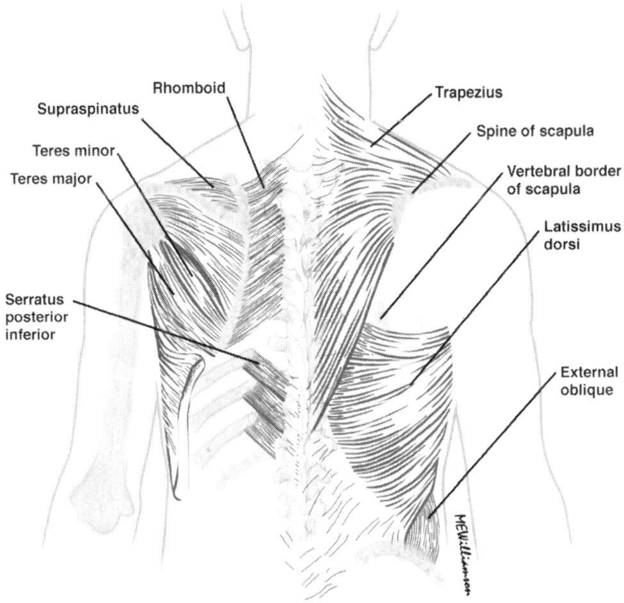

FIG. 1-2. Posterior chest wall anatomy and major muscles of expiration.

Anatomy of the Intercostal Spaces

Each intercostal space is made up of three muscles and a neurovascular bundle that runs between the middle and innermost muscles. The neurovascular bundle (in a caudal direction) is composed of an intercostal vein, intercostal arteries, and an intercostal nerve. In each space lies a single posterior intercostal artery and two anterior intercostal arteries.

The most superficial muscles are the **external intercostal muscles**, which extend downward between the ribs in an anterior direction between the inferior margin of the rib above and the superior aspect of the rib below. The **internal intercostal muscles** are deeper, extending downward in a posterior direction between the subcostal groove of the rib above to the superior border of the rib below. The innermost muscle is the transverse thoracis muscle.

The **anterior intercostal arteries** arise from the internal mammary artery. This artery arises from the subclavian artery and courses caudally down the rib cage approximately 2 cm lateral to the sternum. The anterior intercostal artery divides into a superior and inferior intercostal arterial branch within each intercostal space anteriorly, supplying branches to the parietal pleura, muscles, and skin.

The **posterior intercostal arteries** arise from the subclavian artery and the descending thoracic aorta. Posteriorly they course in the middle of the intercostal space, but pass into the subcostal grove along the lower edge of each rib as they pass along the lateral chest wall.

The **intercostal veins** drain into the azygos or hemiazygos veins posteriorly, and into the internal mammary and musculophrenic veins anteriorly. The **intercostal nerves** provide anterior cutaneous, posterior cutaneous, collateral, and muscular branches, as well as sensory branches to the pleura and peritoneum.

Anatomy of the Lymphatics

The superficial and deep lymphatic networks of the thorax communicate extensively. An efferent trunk draining the costal pleura lies in the intercostal spaces above and below each rib. Posteriorly these drain into lymph nodes along the vertebral column. Anteriorly, these drain into nodes usually found along the 2nd and 3rd intercostal spaces parasternally. Efferent trunks drain from much of the diaphragm and mediastinum to upper mediastinal and tracheobronchial nodes. Lymph drains from these upper nodes into the venous system through communications with the thoracic duct. Some lymph drains from the lower portion of the parietal pleura to retroperitoneal nodes around the kidney.

Anatomy of the Pleural Cavity and Lung

The anatomic pleura consists of a sheet of mesothelial cells that constitutes a translucent membrane. Practically speaking, the pleura also includes adjacent fibrous connective tissue, blood vessels, and lymphatics.

The pleural cavity lies between the visceral pleura, which lines the external surface of the lung, and the parietal pleura, which lines the internal surface of the thoracic cage. The parietal pleura also reflects along the upper surface of the diaphragm and lateral border of the mediastinum. At the hila, it surrounds the pulmonary vessels and bronchi, continuing over the external surface of the lung as the visceral pleura. The **visceral pleura** also reflects along the interlobar fissures so that the pleura covering one lobe is in contact with the visceral pleura of the adjacent lobe.

The parietal pleura is usually smooth and translucent. Ribs, vessels, and muscles are easily seen through the pleural lining. Fat deposits are usually present along the underside of the ribs. Unlike the visceral pleura, the parietal pleura has abundant sensory nerve endings, making it extremely sensitive to touch.

Regions of parietal pleura are usually divided into cervical, costal, diaphragmatic, and mediastinal surfaces for description purposes. The **costodiaphragmatic recess** is the most inferior lying region of the pleural cavity into which the lung expands during deep inspiration. This recess is approximately 3 cm deep anteriorly, 5 cm deep posteriorly, and 8 cm deep laterally.

The lung lies within the pleural cavity. This soft, spongy organ is made up of interstitial tissue and airways. **The right lung** has an upper, middle, and lower lobe, separated by the minor and major fissures (which are infoldings of the visceral pleura). **The left lung** has an upper and lower lobe, separated by the major fissure. The lingula of the upper lobe is an anterior-lying structure and is considered homologous to the middle lobe on the right. The inferior aspects of both lungs lie on the diaphragm. The apex, or superior aspect, of each lung extends above the clavicle into the root of the neck.

The trachea divides into a left and right main bronchus at the carina. Each main bronchus divides into segmental and subsegmental bronchi that eventually feed distal bronchioles and alveoli with air from the atmosphere. In general, there are ten segmental bronchi on the right and nine segmental bronchi on the left.

Basic Physiology and Pleuropulmonary Relationships

The lung usually fills the entire pleural cavity, although it may not fill the small recesses at the cardiophrenic and costophrenic angles. In some cases, small amounts of fluid may be present in these areas.

The fully inflated lung is held against the inner aspect of the rib cage because of apposition between the parietal and visceral pleurae. Usually, only a small amount of pleural fluid (less than 1 mL) is present, acting as a lubricant between the parietal and visceral pleura layers. At functional residual capacity (FRC), this pleural fluid layer is believed to be between 6 and 15 μm thick. FRC is defined as the volume of gas remaining in the lungs at the end of a normal expiration. This volume is usually greater than 3,000 mL in healthy males. An increase in FRC (in which case the thorax is larger than normal) can place the thorax at a mechanical disadvantage, as is seen in the hyperinflated state of the lung in patients with emphysema.

Contact between the lung and chest wall, and therefore between the two pleural surfaces, is maintained because positive atmospheric pressure in the inflated lung keeps it expanded and positive atmospheric pressure outside the thoracic cage is exerted on the chest wall. The lung's natural tendency to collapse is known as **elastic recoil**. If the thoracic cage is open to atmosphere, the lung will collapse because of the elastic recoil, and the chest wall will expand outward because the force of atmospheric pressure on the rib cage is partially lost.

In the closed chest, lung size increases with inspiration (compared to expiration), so that elastic recoil actually increases. With the patient at rest (FRC), the difference between the force of elastic recoil prompting the lung to collapse and the force of the thoracic cage's natural tendency to pull outward creates a negative pressure known as the **pleural pressure**.

Pleural pressure fluctuates with inspiration and expiration, usually becoming more negative with inspiration. Also, there is a **gradient of pleural pressure** of about 0.2 to 0.5 cm H_2O/cm vertical distance, with pleural pressure being most negative in the upper regions of the pleural cavity. In part, this may account for differences in distribution of ventilation in the upper and lower parts of the lung, since alveolar distention may be greater in the upper lobes because of the more negative pleural pressure in this region.

Physiology and Pleural Fluid Movement

The pleura is made up of mesothelial cells, connective tissue, and fibroelastic tissue. Abundant microvillae cover the mesothelial cell surface. Although their function and structure are still uncertain, it appears that microvillae serve to diminish the friction between the lung and the chest wall, transport or secrete enzymes of the pentose and oxidative pathways, synthesize surfactant and glycoproteins, and maintain the integrity of the pleural cavity.

The mesothelial layer is permeable to water, electrolytes, protein, and particles smaller than 4 μm. Electron microscopy has confirmed the existence of **stomas** (pores of Wang) and aggregates of **lymphoid cells** (Kampmeier's foci) that allow communication with vascular and lymphatic channels. Abundant fluid and particulate matter can be removed from the pleural space through the lymphatics.

The pleural space normally contains several milliliters of fluid that serves as a lubricant between pleural surfaces. This fluid is constantly being formed and removed. Any imbalance of factors favoring formation or decreased removal results in an abnormal amount of fluid in the pleural space, thus constituting a **pleural effusion**.

Fluid movement between vascular and extravascular compartments is, for the most part, governed by **Starling's law of**

transcapillary exchange, but also by the permeability of the capillary endothelium. Pleural fluid accumulation occurs from alterations of (1) the filtration coefficient (determines fluid movement through the capillary wall); (2) the colloid osmotic (also known as oncotic) pressure, which is proportional to the protein concentration in the pleural and intravascular fluids; and (3) the hydrostatic pressure (which is the sum of intrapleural and intravascular hydrostatic pressures). Normally, the balance of these forces prevents fluid accumulation in the pleural space.

Fluid movement = filtration coefficient × [(difference between capillary and pleural hydrostatic pressures) – (difference between capillary and pleural oncotic pressures)]

☆ Clinical Pearls

- In the axilla, the second intercostal space is the highest space that can be felt.
- The intercostal space takes its name from the rib above it.
- The pulmonary ligament is a thick portion of parietal pleura that extends between the hilum and the diaphragm. It can be sectioned during thoracotomy to facilitate lung mobilization.
- In pathologic conditions, the amount of fluid may be increased because of decreased absorption or increased secretion of fluid from either pleural surface.
- Normal pleural hydrostatic pressure is approximately –5 cm H_2O. Normal pleural oncotic pressure is approximately +5 cm H_2O.

Heard on the Wards

Question: Do landmarks change when patients are sitting, as for thoracentesis?

Answer: When the shoulders are raised and the arms are folded in front of the patient, the scapulae are pulled outward and above the 6th intercostal space. In the upright sitting position, the diaphragm is approximately at the 8th posterior intercostal space but can be higher in patients with volume loss, ascites, or obesity.

Question: What are the axillary lines?

Answer: Each axillary line extends downward from the axillary folds to the iliac crest. The anterior axillary fold is formed by the lower aspect of the pectoralis major muscle. The posterior axillary fold is formed by the tendon of the latissimus dorsi and lower aspect of the teres major muscle. The midaxillary line runs parallel and vertically downward along the midline between these two folds.

Question: Which muscles control respiration?
Answer: During inspiration the diaphragm contracts. Moving downward, the vertical diameter of the thoracic cage increases. The external intercostal muscles also contract to pull the ribs forward and upward, increasing the anteroposterior and lateral diameters of the thoracic cage. However, if additional ventilation is necessary, or during chronic or acute respiratory failure, accessory respiratory muscles may be recruited to assist in ventilation: the sternocleidomastoid muscles may contract to lift the sternum upward, and the anterior serratus muscles lift the ribs upward. The scalene muscles contract to lift the first two ribs upward, while the pectoralis muscles raise both the ribs and the sternum.

Question: In order to avoid intercostal vessels while performing a thoracentesis, I've been taught to insert the needle along the superior border of the rib that lies just below the chosen intercostal space. I think the saying goes, "above the rib below," right?
Answer: Yes, but remember that posteriorly, there is no internal intercostal muscle, so the bundle lies directly on the parietal pleura, smack dab in the middle of the intercostal space. The neurovascular bundle takes its definitive position under the rib only about 5 to 8 cm lateral to the spine.

Question: What is an exudate?
Answer: Exudates are protein-rich fluids that accumulate in the pleural space primarily because of processes that affect lymphatic drainage and increase vascular permeability (i.e., inflammatory states and neoplasms).

Question: What is a transudate?
Answer: Transudates are protein-poor fluids that accumulate in the pleural space primarily because of processes that alter osmotic and hydrostatic pressures (i.e., heart, liver, or kidney failure) and therefore affect Starling's equation.

Recommended Reading

Agostini E, Zicchi L. Starling forces and lymphatic drainage in pleural liquid and protein exchanges. Respir Physiol 1991;86: 271–281.
A clear description of some very complex processes.

Clemente CD. Anatomy: a regional atlas of the human body. Baltimore: Williams and Wilkins, 1987.

Forster RE, Dubois AB, Briscoe WA, Fisher AB. The lung: physiologic basis of pulmonary function test. Chicago: Year Book Medical, 1986.

Healy JE, Hodge J. Surgical anatomy. Toronto: BC Decker, 1990.
Lots of drawings and a well-written, concise text.

Lai-Fook SJ, Rodarte JR. Pleural pressure distribution and its relationship to lung volume and interstitial pressure. J Appl Physiol 1991;70:967–978.
An excellent review of recent research pertaining to pleural mechanics and the forces that affect pleural fluid movement.

Light RW. Pleural diseases, 3rd ed. Baltimore: Williams and Wilkins, 1995.
A "must-have" reference for any pleural disease specialist. I've had every edition since the first (1983).

Wang NS. Anatomy and physiology of the pleural space. Clin Chest Med 1985;6:3–16.
Includes a concise review of Kampmeier's foci and the pores of Wang.

2. PHYSICAL EXAMINATION OF THE CHEST WALL, LUNGS, AND PLEURA

Signs and Symptoms of Patients with Pleural Disease

Pleuritic chest pain is the most frequent symptom of pleural effusion. Chest discomfort may be acute or gradual in onset. Characteristically, the intensity of the pain increases with inspiration (pleuritic component), radiating to either the abdomen or shoulder, and decreasing with expiration. These symptoms suggest pleural inflammation. Discomfort can also be dull, aching, or throbbing. It usually does not last longer than a few days. Relatively quiet breathing may be associated with grunting during expiration that is related to the patient's attempt to splint the chest.

Dyspnea is often a presenting symptom of the patient with pleural disease. It may be acute or gradual in onset, and usually increases with exertion. Dyspnea often increases when patients are prone or supine. Patients may be unable to lie in the lateral decubitus position, affected side up. Dyspnea can be caused by ineffective ventilation but also by pain from pericardial or pleural inflammation, cardiac disease, or shifting of the mediastinum.

Cough is usually dry and nonproductive. It is often worse at night or when the patient lies supine. The usual antitussives are usually ineffective. Cough can be productive in the case of associated bronchitis or pneumonia. Overall, however, its cause is not well understood.

Fever is often present in a case of infection and may occasionally be present in patients with pulmonary infarction, cancer, or collagen vascular disorders. A low-grade temperature is seen in many patients with pleural tuberculosis.

Other symptoms include chills, shoulder pain, rib pain, abdominal discomfort, nausea or vomiting, chest heaviness or tightness, anxiety, feelings of impending doom, fatigue, weight loss, loss of appetite, arrhythmias, hypoxemia, oxygen desaturation at rest or with exertion, and complaints of **air hunger.**

Physical Examination of Patients with Pleural Disease

A carefully performed **physical examination** is essential in patients with suspected or proven pleural disease. In many instances, it may alleviate the need for costly ancillary examinations such as chest radiography, ultrasound, or computed tomography. The physical examination is best described using the traditional division of inspection, palpation, percussion, and auscultation.

Inspection should be performed with the patient in each of the standing, supine, and seated upright positions. The anterior, lateral, and posterior chest should be examined. Look for abnormal breathing patterns, respiratory rate (breaths per minute), asymmetric chest movements, and sternal retraction. Look for skin lesions, subcutaneous lumps and bumps, increased venous or capillary filling, as well as grunting during respiration, splinting during deep inspiration, increased abdominal breathing, or a desire to lie on the affected side. The following **anatomic landmarks** should be noted (Figs. 2-1 and 2-2):

- The male **nipple** is approximately at the level of the 4th intercostal space (corresponding to the 4th thoracic vertebra).

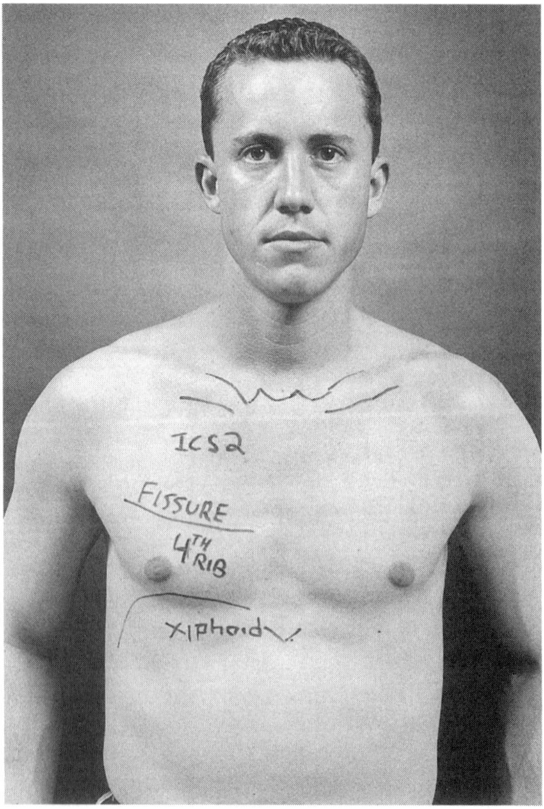

FIG. 2-1. Anatomic landmarks of the anterior chest.

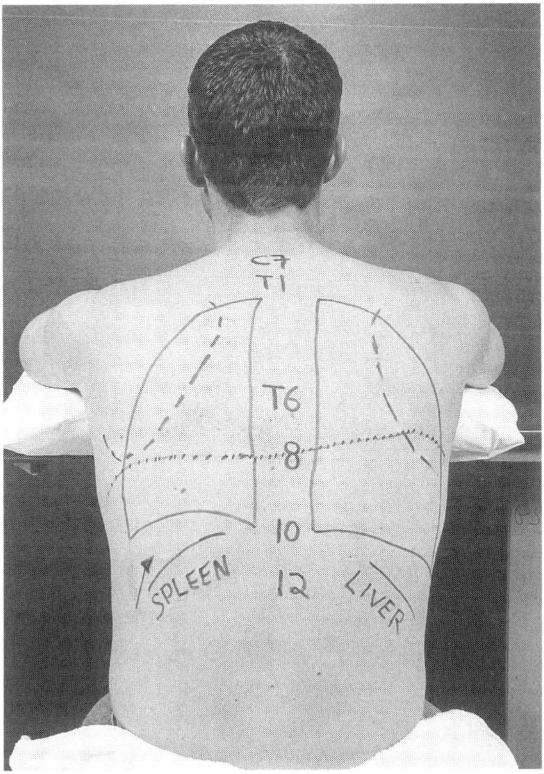

FIG. 2-2. Anatomic landmarks of the posterior chest.

- The inferior **angle of the scapula** is approximately level with the spine of the 7th or 8th thoracic vertebra.
- The lower tip of the **scapula** lies approximately at the level of the 6th intercostal space in the seated patient, arms held forward and shoulders raised.
- The **major fissure** extends obliquely downward and laterally from the root of the spine of the scapula (approximately the 3rd thoracic vertebra) to the 6th costochondral junction, crossing the midaxillary line at approximately the 4th intercostal space on the right and the 5th intercostal spacc on the left.
- On inspection of the lateral chest, the anterior, mid-, and posterior **axillary lines** are defined by a line drawn between the uppermost aspect of the pectoralis major in the axilla and the anterior iliac crest (anterior axillary line), the midaxilla and superior aspect of the iliac crest

(midaxillary line), and the uppermost aspect of the latissimus dorsi in the axilla and the posterior aspect of the iliac crest (posterior axillary line) (Fig. 2-3).

Palpation is best performed with the patient sitting, shoulders raised and hunched forward to pull the scapula superiorly and laterally. Using the same hand, test for tactile fremitus by placing only the palmar surface of the hand on the chest while asking the patient to say "ninety-nine." Compare the upper, middle, and lower portions of each hemithorax sequentially to ascertain symmetry or differences. Start from the top and work downward. The intercostal spaces should be counted using the following **landmarks**:

- The anteromedial aspect of the **2nd intercostal space** is located by palpating the head of the 2nd rib at the angle of Louis, located at the junction between the manubrium and body of the sternum.
- The 2nd intercostal space is also the highest space that can be felt during palpation of the **axilla**.
- Along the midaxillary line, **the 10th rib** is the most inferiorly rib that can be felt. More posteriorly, the 11th and 12th "floating" ribs are easily palpable in thin patients.

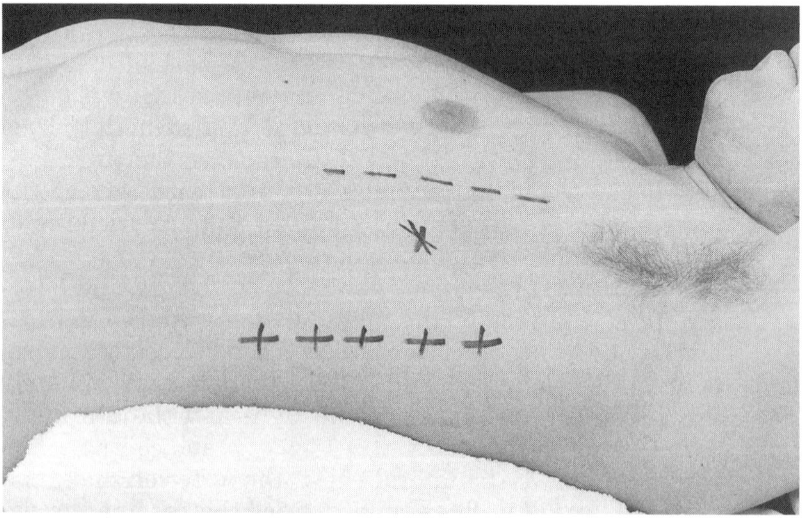

FIG. 2-3. Lateral chest wall showing anterior (–), mid- (*), and posterior (++) axillary lines, and positioning for chest tube insertion through the 5th intercostal space (*).

Percussion is best performed with the patient sitting, shoulders raised and hunched forward to pull the scapula superiorly and laterally. Indirect (two-handed manual) percussion is best performed by placing the distal extremities of one's medius or index finger on the chest and lightly striking it with the tip of the flexed index finger of the other hand. The wrist should be loose and relaxed. The elbow and shoulder are not participating in the maneuver. The striking finger should simply bounce off the resting finger. Several strikes may be necessary before displacing the resting finger to a lower aspect on the chest wall. The upper, middle, and lower aspects of each hemithorax are thus examined sequentially to detect asymmetry or percussion abnormalities. Start from the top and work downward. The normal, air-filled lung is resonant, except for the areas of cardiac (2nd to 6th intercostal space on the left midclavicular line) and hepatic dullness anteriorly (4th to 6th intercostal space on the right midclavicular line). Remember that

- The **left and right hemidiaphragm** are relatively symmetric. At the end of a normal expiration, the dome of each hemidiaphragm rests approximately at the 5th intercostal space anteriorly, and at the 8th intercostal space posteriorly in the erect patient.
- **The liver**, lying below the diaphragm, may extend as high as the 4th intercostal space on the right and the 5th intercostal space on the left during forced expiration.

Auscultation will elicit normal, diminished, abnormal, or absent breath sounds. Listen for fine crackles, coarse crackles, wheezing, and rhonchi. Ask yourself whether crackles or rhonchi disappear or increase after coughing; and whether abnormal sounds are heard during inspiration or expiration. Examine each hemithorax sequentially, starting from the top. Listen for a pleural friction rub (inconstant, coarse, leathery sounds) during late deep inspiration or early expiration.

Physical Findings in Patients with Pleural Effusions

Inspection

The hemithorax may be enlarged and the intercostal spaces expanded in the case of abundant pleural fluid and contralateral shift of the mediastinum. The hemithorax may be retracted and the intercostal spaces may be narrowed in the case of volume loss, trapped lung, or ipsilateral shift of the mediastinum. The usual concavity of the intercostal spaces may be lost or appear to bulge or expand in the case of a large effusion.

Palpation
The intercostal spaces may be enlarged or narrowed. There may be tenderness over the ribs (particularly in the case of metastatic bone disease or rib fractures). Tactile fremitus is absent or diminished on the affected side. Maximum cardiac impulse may be shifted to the side opposite the effusion (in this case, the contralateral side is the right) in the case of a large unilateral left-sided effusion.

Percussion
Dullness is usually greatest at the bases. A shifting area of dullness with change of body position is virtually pathognomonic.

Auscultation
Breath sounds are absent or diminished. A pleural rub (an inconstant coarse, leathery sound) may be heard toward the end of a deep inspiration or during early expiration. Egophony (described as a nasal or bleating quality to spoken syllables) may be heard above the level of the effusion but is impaired by compressed lung below the level of the effusion.

Physical Findings in Patients with Pneumothorax

Inspection
The hemithorax may be enlarged and the intercostal spaces expanded, particularly in the case of large pneumothorax with contralateral shift of the mediastinum. Ipsilateral respiratory excursion may be diminished.

Palpation
The intercostal spaces may be enlarged. Rib fractures may be felt. Tactile fremitus is absent or diminished on the affected side. In the case of tension pneumothorax, the trachea and mediastinal structures may be shifted to the contralateral side.

Percussion
Resonance or hyperresonance on the affected side.

Auscultation
Breath sounds are absent or diminished on the affected side.

☆ Clinical Pearls

- After removing the patient's shirt or blouse, take a few minutes to observe the patient's breathing pattern and note anatomic landmarks.
- For tactile fremitus, only the palmar surface of the hand should touch the chest wall.

- For indirect chest percussion, only the distal phalange of the medius or index finger should touch the chest wall. The striking finger should be firmly flexed, and the strike should be made using the natural force of the flexed wrist, not the arm.
- The disappearance of diaphragmatic excursion on the involved side is known as Litten's sign.
- When pain is transmitted from the diaphragm to a spot on the ipsilateral shoulder, patients will usually point to the spot, classically known as Capp's point.
- Miscellaneous signs and symptoms associated with illnesses that cause pleural disease include (1) neck vein distension in the upright position; a tender, enlarged liver; or pedal edema suggestive of congestive heart failure; (2) dilated veins over the anterior chest suggestive of superior vena cava syndrome from cancer or vascular thromboembolic disease; (3) large, nontender liver with nodular hepatic metastases; (4) joint deformities, subcutaneous nodules, or dermatologic findings suggestive of rheumatoid arthritis or connective tissue disorders; (5) ascites and pelvic tumor suggestive of Meigs' syndrome; (6) nipple retraction or nodules noted on breast exam suggestive of breast cancer; and (7) palpable lymph nodes or splenomegaly suggestive of lymphoma or leukemia.

Heard on the Wards

Question: How do I count the intercostal spaces?
Answer: Use your fingers. The second intercostal space is the highest space you can feel in the axilla along the midaxillary line.

Question: How do I describe breath sounds?
Answer: Concisely. Everyone should understand what you are describing. The words fine and coarse crackles, rhonchi, and wheezes, therefore, are far better than the vague "rales" so often heard on the wards.

Question: Are pulmonary function tests warranted in patients with pleural effusions or thickening?
Answer: Patients with pleural thickening may have restrictive ventilatory impairment. Incremental exercise testing may also be warranted to determine degree of breathlessness and potential disability (resulting from an empyema-related pleural peel

or asbestos-related pleuropulmonary disease, for example). Patients with effusions may have decreased maximum inspiratory or expiratory pressures, restrictive ventilatory impairment, and occasionally expiratory flow obstruction. Complete drainage of the effusion, therefore, is warranted before testing.

Recommended Reading

DeGowin RL. DeGowin and DeGowin's bedside diagnostic examination. New York: Macmillan, 1987.

A classic text, although a bit heavy to carry around in your coat pocket.

3. RADIOLOGY OF THE PLEURA

✣ Definition

Pleural radiology is the study of pleuropulmonary and chest wall relationships using appropriately selected imaging techniques to localize pleural abnormalities. Imaging studies have become indispensable in the modern care of patients with pleural disease, and they are particularly valuable for detecting small effusions or air in the pleural space as well as to guide thoracentesis or chest tube insertion.

■ Basic Principles

Standard radiographic techniques include frontal posteroanterior and lateral, oblique, and recumbent chest radiographs. **Conventional frontal and lateral chest radiographs** usually suffice to detect pleural abnormalities and coexistent lung parenchymal disease. Lateral views will often demonstrate effusions before they are evident on frontal views because the lowest part of the pleural space is posterior and inferior. Fluid, therefore, accumulates there first. In some cases, small amounts of fluid may also be noted as a wedge of increased density in the major interlobar fissure. **Oblique views** increase the likelihood of detecting plaques and extrapleural fat. The side of the patient (left or right) touching the cassette holder determines the side of the view. **Recumbent views,** also referred to as lateral decubitus views, are helpful for distinguishing free-flowing fluid from loculated effusions. Small amounts of pleural fluid not readily seen on supine views (100 mL or less) may be detected as layering of the fluid along the dependent lateral chest wall by cross-table radiography.

Computed tomography (CT) provides cross-sectional, two-dimensional images that overcome the problems caused by superimposition of anatomic structures seen with chest radiographs. Particularly useful to assess the extent of pleural thickening, tumor invasion, and degree of pulmonary or extrapleural disease, CT scans are usually obtained in the supine position during full inspiration. CT is unreliable in determining the amount of pleural carcinomatosis, especially if lesions are small, nodular, and diffuse. Limited scans may be useful to study a focal area of pleural abnormality. Intravenous injection of noniodinated contrast material may facilitate interpretation of complex pleuropulmonary abnormalities and visualization of vascular structures. Digital image reconstruction using contrast, spatial, multiplanar, or three-dimensional volume rendering can improve visualization of anatomic detail.

Magnetic resonance imaging (MRI) is based on the principle that atomic nuclei re-emit absorbed energy delivered by radiowaves of certain frequencies. It is most useful to define complex pleuropulmonary relationships and evaluate chest wall or mediastinal invasion because of its high tissue differentiation capabilities and capacity for superb visualization of vascular structures. Its role, however, is limited because image quality is adversely affected by respiratory motion and the heterogeneous structure (air and tissue) of the lung. Although no radiation is delivered, the magnetic field required can modify pacemaker function and is contraindicated in patients with metal clips near the eye or spinal cord.

❍ Indications

- To identify pathologic processes roentgenologically. These may include pleural effusions, pneumothorax, pleural-based masses, mediastinal adenopathy of tumors, postsurgical changes, and pulmonary parenchymal diseases including but not limited to pneumonia, interstitial lung disease, pleuropulmnonary infections, inflammatory diseases and vasculitis, pulmonary vascular disease, and cancer.
- Radiologic imaging studies are often warranted in patients with known extrathoracic or systemic illnesses in order to detect associated thoracic or cardiac involvement, chest wall abnormalities, or diaphragmatic dysfunction, as well as in asymptomatic individuals as part of routine screening programs.
- To help correlate roentgenologic findings with clinical setting in order to establish a differential diagnosis and assist in decisions pertaining to medical and surgical management decisions or the need for diagnostic or therapeutic procedures.

● Contraindications

- There are no contraindications to these imaging studies although proper shielding precautions should be taken in pregnant women.
- Contrast material should be avoided in patients with allergies to dyes or other contrast agents, as well as in selected patients with renal dysfunction. Premedication with corticosteroids and antihistamines is often warranted. Screening for allergies, renal insufficiency, or a history of

adverse events has become a standard component of the preimaging assessment in most radiology departments.

- Patients with severe claustrophobia are often unable to undergo CT or MRI scanning. General anesthesia in these cases may be necessary if the procedure is absolutely warranted.
- Patients with metal clips should avoid MRI because the magnetic field may cause migration of recently placed surgical clips, aneurysmal clips, or metal projections in the eyes.

❖ Equipment and Techniques

A detailed description of imaging equipment and techniques is beyond the scope of this manual. The expert interpreter of radiographic imaging studies, however, is equipped with a thorough knowledge of anatomy and has developed the technical expertise to formulate a differential diagnosis based on both the imaging findings and the clinical setting. It is always helpful, therefore, to provide clinical information to the radiologists or clinicians interpreting the imaging study because this will help them formulate a differential diagnosis. The following paragraphs are designed to help nonradiologists improve their basic skills at interpreting imaging studies.

Normal Radiographic Pleural Anatomy

The visceral pleural lining of the lung is usually in contact with the parietal pleural lining of the chest wall. Despite this combined thickness, usually less than 1 mm, the pleura is invisible radiographically, except at the interlobar fissures, where **pleural reflections** are outlined on both sides by air-filled lung parenchyma.

Fissures are often seen on conventional chest radiographs as thin, single or double lines approximately 0.2 mm thick. On the lateral view, right and left oblique fissures are differentiated by the continuity of the left fissure to the left hemidiaphragm over the **gastric air bubble,** or the right hemidiaphragm over the liver. CT identification of fissures is essential to proper localization of both pleural and lung parenchymal abnormalities. Their appearance is variable, depending on their axis relative to the plane and the thickness of the cross-section. The left and right **major fissures** (i.e., oblique) appear as broad, avascular bands within the lung parenchyma on conventional 1-cm slices, but they may show as lines on 1-mm slices. The minor fissure on the right appears as an ovoid or triangular avascular band (Fig. 3-1).

The left and right **pulmonary ligaments** are reflections of the mediastinal parietal pleura extending from the inferior margin of the hilum toward the diaphragm, like the dependent part of a

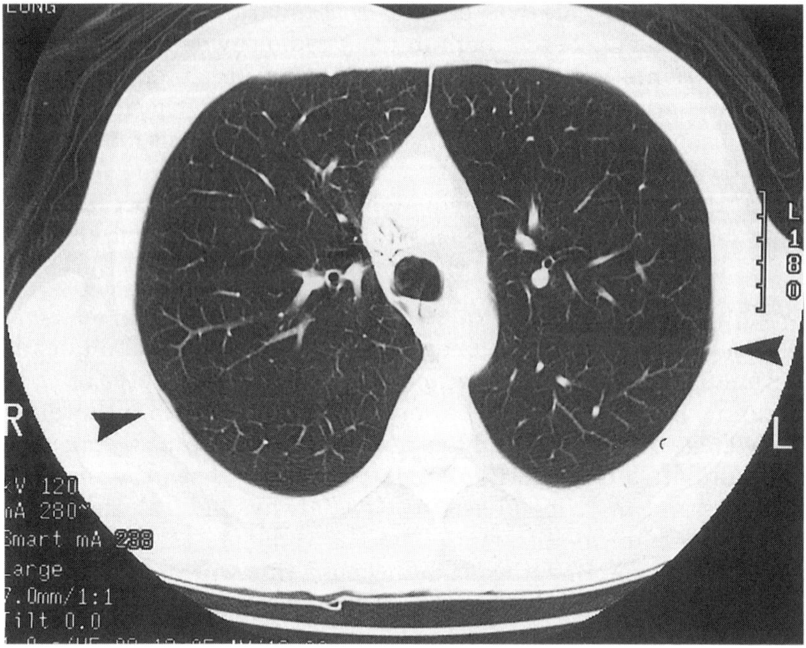

FIG. 3-1. A computed tomography scan using 7-mm sections at the level of the lower trachea shows a normal major fissure on the right visible as a broad avascular band within lung parenchyma *(arrowhead).* The major fissure on the left is visible as a thin line *(arrowhead).*

sleeve. Rarely seen on conventional chest radiographs, the pulmonary ligaments are often visible on CT scans, where they appear as thin triangular bands between the medial aspect of the hemidiaphragm and the mediastinum, in close proximity to the esophagus on the left and the inferior vena cava on the right.

The **chest wall** is well visualized on conventional radiographs and CT scans. Companion shadows caused by tangential projections of the horizontal x-ray beam on visceral and parietal pleural surfaces and intrapleural or extrapleural fat should not be confused with the visceral pleural line of a pneumothorax, particularly at the apex. On chest radiographs, **ribs** are counted from top to bottom, anterior separately from posterior. On CT scans, the anterior aspect of the first rib is identified and subsequent ribs are counted posteriorly along the rib cage on sequential images.

Describing Radiographic Abnormalities

Gravitational forces cause **fluid** to accumulate in dependent areas. As fluid collects between the inferior aspect of the lung and the hemidiaphragm, it may accumulate in the posterior, lateral, or anterior portions of the costophrenic sinus, eventually obliterating the costophrenic angle. As fluid accumulates, the lung retracts while maintaining its original shape. Thus, the miniaturized lung floats on a layer of fluid which appears on posteroanterior chest radiographs as a homogeneous opacity with a meniscus-shaped, concave upper border higher laterally than medially. In reality, the level of fluid is horizontal, and the meniscus-shaped projection is caused by the increased radiodensity to the x-ray beam as it passes through a greater amount of fluid laterally than medially.

Air, on the other hand, rises to the highest point in the hemithorax unless entrapped within a fissure or between pleuropulmonary adhesions. In the posteroanterior view, air collections are most readily seen in the upper third of the hemithorax. As the lung retracts inward, a visceral pleural line becomes visible because it is outlined by air-filled lung parenchyma on one side and by the air-filled pleural cavity on the other. The radiodensity of the collapsing lung parenchyma does not change until substantial atelectasis occurs (Fig. 3-2).

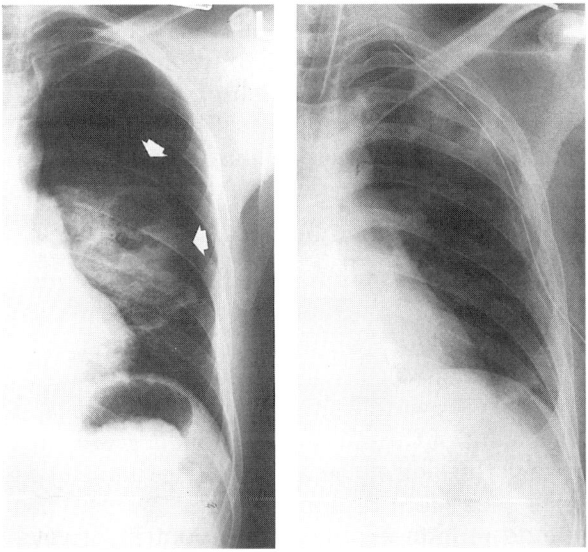

FIG. 3-2. Patient with AIDS and pneumothorax from ruptured pneumocyst. Posteroanterior chest radiographs show visceral pleural line adjacent to ruptured pneumocyst *(arrows)* and large-bore chest tube placed in appropriate position in the apex.

Parietal and visceral **pleural abnormalities** should be described in terms of their

- Shape (round, squared-off, convex, concave, meniscus-like).
- Radiodensity (lucent or opaque) and margins (smooth or irregular).
- Appearance (pseudotumoral, nodular, mass-like, plaque).
- Size (small, moderate, or large) and extent (uni- or bilateral, focal or diffuse).
- Location (across fissures or confined to a single lobe, or involving a portion of the hemithorax, posterior, anterior, or lateral costal and diaphragmatic parietal pleural, or visceral pleura).
- Effect on the hemidiaphragm (obliteration, elevation, inversion, change in contour).
- Presence of coexistent pulmonary or chest wall abnormalities (invasion, fractures, masses, infiltrates, atelectasis, consolidation).

Pleural effusions may be described as **free-flowing** or loculated, in which case they may be encapsulated by adhesions or firm juxtapositions of visceral and parietal pleura, or accumulate within folds of lung parenchyma or within the fissures themselves (intralobar effusion). Sometimes, fluid takes on the appearance of a pseudotumor: in lateral projections, loculated effusions within a fissure tend to have bulges on both sides. **Loculations** also occur between the lung and chest wall, as fluid becomes encapsulated by fibrinous or fibrotic adhesions, usually of inflammatory origin. These pleural opacities are usually smooth and broad-based.

Pleural Effusions

Large pleural effusions may have a mass effect, causing inversion of the diaphragm, mediastinal shift to the contralateral side, or even complete "white-out" of the hemithorax. Diaphragmatic inversion occurs most frequently on the left side, causing concavity upward of the hemidiaphragm and a downward displacement of the gastric air bubble. A shift of the mediastinum toward the side of the fluid, rather than the usual direction, suggests that pleural pressures are lower on the involved side and should prompt evaluation for **central airways obstruction**, usually from bronchogenic carcinoma or tracheobronchial metastases.

Small effusions may be subpulmonic or may fill only the costophrenic or cardiophrenic sinuses. **Subpulmonic effusions**

are suspected if one or both hemidiaphragms appear elevated, if the distance between the gastric air bubble and the superior margin of the left hemidiaphragm (usually less than 2 cm) is increased, or if the highest point on the presumed hemidiaphragm is more lateral than normal, especially on the right (Fig. 3-3).

Pleural Thickening and Fibrosis

Pleural thickening can result from neoplasms (lymphoma, metastatic carcinoma, and mesothelioma), inflammatory or infectious diseases (tuberculosis, fungal diseases, sarcoidosis, pleurisy, empyema), trauma, hemothorax, collagen vascular diseases, and industrial or occupational exposures (asbestos, talc, berylliosis, silicosis). Late **calcifications** are not uncommon, and extensive pleural **fibrosis** can result in restrictive lung disease. Although pleural thickening can be seen on conventional chest radiographs, the CT scan is best to delineate its extent.

Calcified **hyaline plaques** are recognized tangentially as radiopaque, well-defined, elevated linear structures, usually

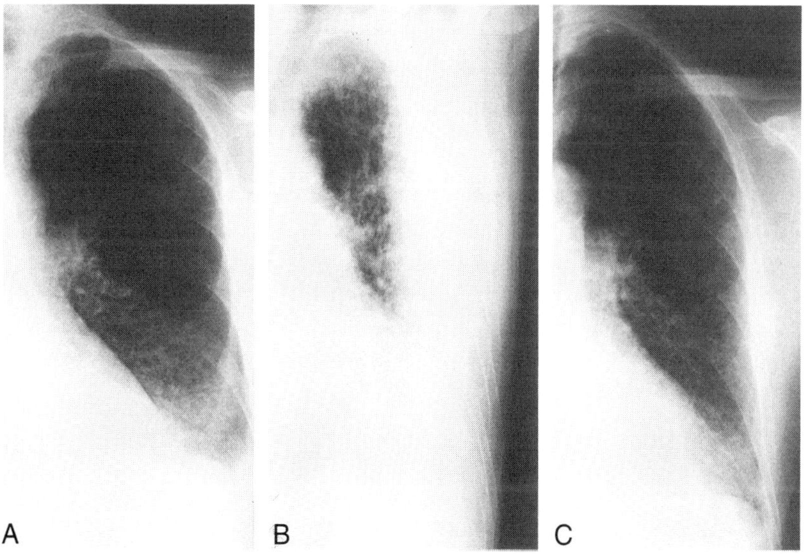

FIG. 3-3. Large subpulmonic effusion with blunting of costophrenic angle **(A)**. Left lateral decubitus view demonstrates layering of fluid along lateral chest wall **(B)**. Pleural effusion has been evacuated as demonstrated on postthoracentesis chest radiograph **(C)**. A substantial amount of fluid may be hidden in the subpulmonic area.

located on the diaphragm and posterolateral costal pleural surfaces. When calcified, plaques appear tangentially as linear stripes of density, notably on the diaphragm, where there is no soft tissue component seen. Small plaques are usually parallel to the ribs, but larger plaques will bridge the intercostal spaces, forming large pancake-like structures. **Extrapleural fat** is similar to plaques in distribution and, like them, spares the costophrenic angle. **Diffuse pleural fibrosis**, on the other hand, is usually recognized as smooth, continuous thickening of a large portion of the conjoined visceral and parietal pleural surfaces, often with associated expansion of extrapleural fat, as seen on CT.

Solitary or diffuse **pleural nodules** are seen in malignant mesothelioma, benign fibrous mesothelioma, pleural carcinomatosis, superior sulcus tumors, benign tumors such as lipomas or amyloid, pleural sarcomas, Kaposi's sarcoma, and lymphoma. Usually apparent as a raised, dense pleural abnormality, distinction from intrapulmonary lesions can be difficult. CT scans and MRI help delineate the extent of abnormalities and potential invasion of the chest wall, lung, or other contiguous structures (Fig. 3-4).

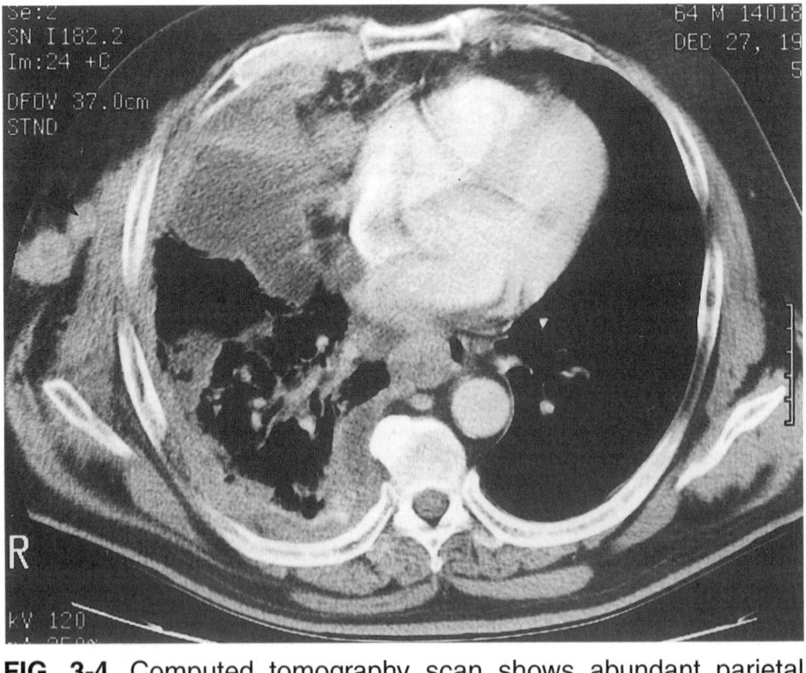

FIG. 3-4. Computed tomography scan shows abundant parietal pleural thickening and tumor from malignant pleural mesothelioma of right hemithorax, also invading the chest wall and muscles.

Pneumothorax

Pneumothoraces are described as small, moderate, or large. These are usually subjective assessments because precise measurement of the size of a pneumothorax is very imprecise in view of the tridimensionality of the lung. They may be spontaneous and idiopathic (as in asthenic young men), iatrogenic (after an invasive procedure such as thoracentesis or central line placement), or secondary (from ruptured blebs or bullae in patients with emphysema, for example).

Free air in the pleural space is easily recognized when the visceral pleural line is demonstrated on upright posteroanterior chest films. Examining a dark film with a **bright light** is helpful. A small pneumothorax can be more easily seen on a decubitus film using a horizontal ray beam because the air rises to the lateral chest wall, and is thus unobscured by the bony and vascular structures of the apex. **Expiratory films** are not so useful as traditionally described, but the difficulty of detecting a pneumothorax should not be underestimated (Fig. 3-5).

A **hydropneumothorax** (defined as both air and fluid in the pleural space) is usually represented as a straight **air-fluid level** within the pleural space (straight as in parallel to the surface of

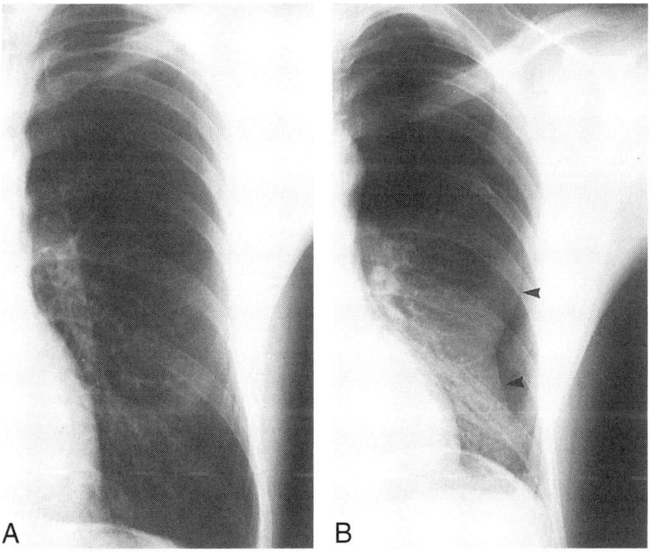

FIG. 3-5. Spontaneous pneumothorax almost invisible in inspiratory view **(A)** but is more clearly visible in expiratory view **(B)** *(arrowheads)*.

the earth). Causes include effusions associated with uncomplicated pneumothoraces, inadvertent air entry during thoracentesis or closed-needle pleural biopsy, chest trauma, thoracic surgery with lung resection, a trapped or incompletely expanded lung, esophageal rupture, and rupture of tuberculous or other infectious cavities and abscesses. Hydropyopneumothoraces are frequently loculated (Fig. 3-6).

Lung Abscess and Empyema

Differentiating between a **lung abscess** and a **bronchopleural fistula** can be difficult. Sterile and infected empyemas accompany pneumonia, appearing much like any other fluid collection. Loculations are common. Secondary collapse of the lower lobe is seen with large effusions. Indeed, it may be difficult to distinguish secondary lobar collapse from lobar consolidation with a small effusion. A bacterial **empyema** may be associated with a lung abscess or, even more likely, with a necrotizing pneumonia (such as staphylococcal), which can go on to form a bronchopleural fistula.

Differentiating Pleural Abnormalities from Parenchymal or Extrapleural Disease

CT scans and MRI are more helpful than chest radiographs. **Extrapleural lesions** usually displace overlying pleura, resulting in an obtuse angle between the lesion and the chest wall. **Pleural**

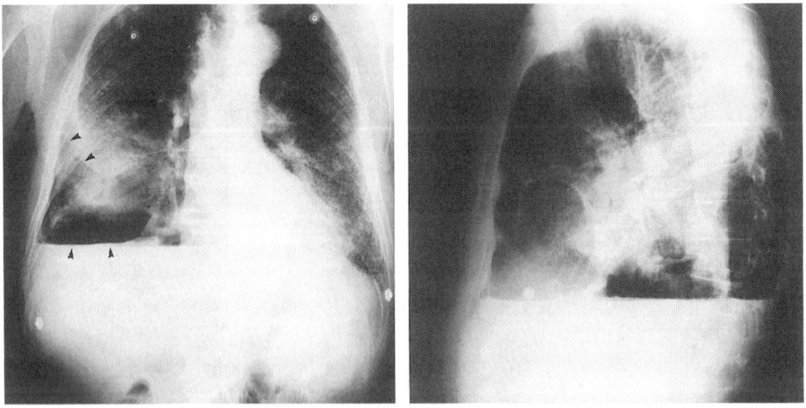

FIG. 3-6. Posteroanterior and lateral views of hydropneumothorax in a patient with coccidioidomycosis empyema and secondary pneumothorax. Note collapsed lung and visceral pleural line *(upper arrowheads)*, as well as straight fluid level denoting fluid in pleural space *(lower arrowheads)*.

lesions are often confined to the pleura, also causing obtuse angles. Appearance is altered, however, by the shape, extent of invasion, adhesions, and adjacent pleural thickening or fluid. **Parenchymal lesions** abut the pleura, causing acute angles between the lesion and the chest wall, although appearance is altered by the lesion's size, extent of pleural invasion, and adjacent pulmonary abnormalities (Fig. 3-7).

▼ Complications

- Adverse reactions to contrast material may include rash, respiratory distress, renal failure, and even death. These can be avoided by proper screening and use of premedication.
- The confined space of a CT or MRI scanner can cause high-grade anxiety, fear, tachypnea, and exacerbated feelings of claustrophobia. Problems are often avoided by careful explanation of the procedure, by administration of short-acting anxiolytics, and by providing patients with a relaxed, cheerful, but professional atmosphere in the imaging suite.
- Central lines, supplemental oxygen, or even tubing to mechanical ventilators may be inadvertently disconnected

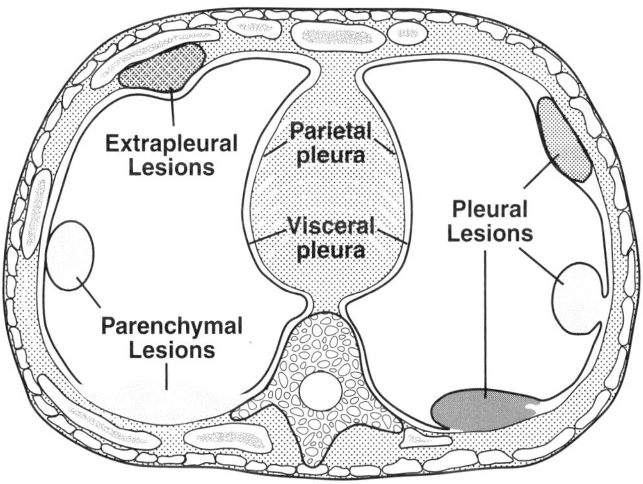

FIG. 3-7. Cross-section of typical and atypical pleural, extrapleural, and peripheral lung parenchymal lesions. Pleural lesions often form obtuse angles between the lesion and the chest wall, although acute angles may be formed when lesions are pedunculated. Parenchymal lesions often form acute angles with the chest wall. Pleural fibrosis, thickening, or loculated fluid formations may cause fusion of visceral and parietal pleural surfaces, often mimicking tumor.

during positioning for bedside chest radiographs. This is easily avoided by assuring proper radiology technician training and providing diligent nursing and respiratory therapist care.

☆ Clinical Pearls

- If fluid (which is radiopaque) or air (which is radiolucent) is interposed between the visceral and parietal pleural surfaces, the lung retracts inward, maintaining its overall shape regardless of the extent of collapse. However, the lung will tend toward localized collapse in case of limited pleural space–occupying lesions. The functional separation of the superior segment and the basal segments of the lower lobe predisposes to separate collapse. Collapse can also be localized if pleuropulmonary adhesions are present.
- Radiographic signs of asbestos-related pleuropulmonary disease include diffuse or localized pleural thickening, rounded atelectasis, calcified and uncalcified hyaline pleural plaques, and benign exudative effusions.
- Lamellar effusions are small effusions tracking along the lateral chest wall, usually forming a sharp angle with the diaphragm. These small effusions show that blunting of the costophrenic angle is not essential to make a diagnosis of pleural fluid. On the other hand, blunting of this angle by slips of the diaphragm in chronic obstructive pulmonary disease show that it does not define pleural fluid either.
- Fluid in the major fissure gives a hazy veil over the lower lobe. It is often interrupted medially by a round lucency, which turns out to be continuous lung across an incomplete fissure. This should not be mistaken for a pneumatocele or bulla.
- Skin folds can be erroneously confused with a thickened visceral pleural line suggestive of pneumothorax. Folds can be distinguished from visceral pleura because they are usually thick and cross anatomic boundaries such as fissures, and are crossed by vascular shadows.
- Tension physiology (with contralateral displacement of the mediastinum, tachycardia, hypotension, dyspnea, and risk of death) can occur from pneumothorax. Air has entered the pleural space and cannot be evacuated during expiration (this is also known as a ball-valve effect of a bronchopleural fistula). Eventually, intrapleural pressure becomes increasingly positive, prompting the contralateral

shift. Emergent thoracentesis and chest tube drainage is curative.

Heard on the Wards

Question: What is the most frequently noted abnormality of malignant mesothelioma?

Answer: Diffuse involvement of the pleural surface by tumor, usually associated with a large effusion, is the hallmark of malignant mesothelioma. In practice, however, it is more likely that pleural carcinomatosis with an adenocarcinoma is the culprit, since it is a more common lesion.

Question: Are there typical appearances of pleural effusions?

Answer: Typical appearance of a pleural effusions can actually be quite subtle, represented as a hazy obliteration of the costophrenic angle. Between 100 and 250 cm^3 of fluid are usually necessary to fill this potential space. As the amount of fluid increases, an upward concavity appears. With sufficient fluid, the density is confluent with the diaphragm.

Question: What about atypical appearances of pleural effusions?

Answer: Atypical appearances of pleural effusions are often noted when fluid accumulates in the interlobar fissures, or when loculated effusions are confined to the outer margins of the lung and pleural space because of adhesions. A localized effusion is often sharply outlined, with rounded margins whose base lies at the periphery. An opaque convexity points inward toward the lung due to the compressibility of the lung by the loculated fluid. Anterior mediastinal effusions are seen as ribbon-shaped shadows parallel to the cardiac silhouette producing a double cardiac contour. Posterior mediastinal effusions are seen as ribbon-shaped shadows parallel to the left or right of the vertebral column, or as triangular shadows within the costophrenic angle.

Question: What is rounded atelectasis?

Answer: Also known as folded lung, rounded atelectasis is a common manifestation of asbestos-related pleuropulmonary disease. Usually, a posteriorly and inferiorly located pleural-based density is noted on a chest radiograph. The CT scan reveals a peripheral wedge-shaped lung mass, toward which curve bronchi and vessels adjacent to an area of focal parietal pleural thickening. Rounded atelectasis is thought to be caused by localized compressive atelectasis and infolding of lung parenchyma adjacent to an area of extensive visceral pleural fibrosis.

Question: When should I consider ordering lateral decubitus films?

Answer: These films are helpful to localize small volumes of pleural fluid (less than 100 mL), demonstrate positional changes in air-fluid levels, or visualize a small pneumothorax. The patient is placed on one side (usually the dependent hemithorax is the one being examined), and the x-ray beam is oriented horizontally. Free-flowing fluid will be seen accumulating along the lateral rib cage in the most dependent areas. Remember that in this position if the dependent hemidiaphragm is elevated its excursion is increased.

Question: Can all pleural plaques be visualized radiographically?

Answer: No. Seen from straight on (en face), calcified plaques appear irregular. Uncalcified plaques, especially along the costal wall, are difficult to detect.

Question: How do I differentiate bronchopleural fistula and a lung abscess?

Answer: Differentiating between a lung abscess and a bronchopleural fistula (BPF) is difficult. The first step is to recognize the fluid level, which requires an upright or decubitus radiograph made with a horizontal ray beam. Next, check the proximity of the abnormality to the ribs and ensure that the entire wall of the pocket is well defined. Finally, check the cross-sectional dimensions of the collection. A lung abscess is not likely to be next to the chest wall, its entire abscess wall is seen and its cross-section is roughly circular. A BPF pocket is right next to the ribs (unless there has been pneumonia for some time), may not have a superior margin, and its horizontal cross-section is elliptical or parallel to the potential space of the pleura. The most common location for a BPF is posterior, so it must also be distinguished from iatrogenic air in the pleural space.

Question: What is the difference between blebs and bullae?

Answer: Blebs are intrapleural or subpleural collections of air usually 1 cm or less in diameter. Overlying pleura is usually translucent, and no trabecular structure is seen. Bullae, on the other hand, are defined as marked focal dilatations of airspaces resulting from the coalescence of adjacent areas of emphysema. Trabecular structure is often maintained.

Recommended Reading

Felson B. Chest roentgenology. Philadelphia: WB Saunders, 1973.
A "must-read" for anyone interested in pleural or pulmonary diseases.

Fraser RG, Pare JAP, Pare PD, Fraser RS, Genereux GP. Diagnosis of diseases of the chest, 3rd ed. Philadelphia: WB Saunders, 1990.
Great text (four volumes) and wonderful images.

Friedman PJ, Hellekant CA. Radiologic recognition of bronchopleural fistula. Radiology 1977;124:289–295.
A nice description of radiographic findings.

Hughson WG, Friedman PJ, Feigin DS, Resnik R, Moser KM. Postpartum pleural effusion: a common radiologic finding. Ann Intern Med 1982;97:856–858.
Still a classic.

Kreel L. Radiology of the pleura. In: Chretian J, Bignon J, Hirsch A, eds. The pleura in health and disease. Lung biology in health and disease, vol 30. New York: Marcel Dekker, 1985: 643–693.
A well-written chapter of an excellent book.

Naidich DP, Zerhouni EA, Siegelman SS. Computed tomography and magnetic resonance of the thorax. New York: Raven Press, 1991.
A superb explanation of CT and MRI interpretation with concise legends and perfectly clear images.

4. ULTRASONOGRAPHY OF THE PLEURA

✤ Definition

Ultrasound is a wave of acoustic energy traveling through a solid, liquid, or gas medium with a frequency greater than the upper limit of human hearing (20,000 Hz).

■ Basic Principles

Sound waves are described by their **frequency** (the number of cycles of an acoustic variable that occur in 1 second), **period** (the time it takes to complete one cycle, typically microseconds), **amplitude** (the magnitude of the sound wave, usually in decibels), **intensity** (the power of the sound beam divided by its cross-sectional area, usually in watts per square centimeter), **wavelength** (the distance occupied by one cycle, usually 0.1 to 0.8 mm in soft tissues), propagation speed (also known as the **acoustic velocity**, or speed at which the sound travels through the medium, typically expressed in meters per second), and **attenuation** (the weakening of the sound wave as it travels through the medium, often reported in negative decibels) (Fig. 4-1).

A **transducer** converts electrical energy to acoustic energy during transmission and acoustic energy to electric energy during reception due to a **piezoelectric crystal** that changes shape and vibrates when the electric current is applied. A damping element (usually made of epoxy resin) is bonded to the back of the crystal, improving image quality and allowing the crystal to react to the returning sound wave. Because air scatters sound, a gel interface is necessary between the transducer and the skin to establish **acoustic coupling**.

Pleural ultrasound data are usually displayed as a **B-mode** (brightness), gray scale, sagittal section of the target. After the

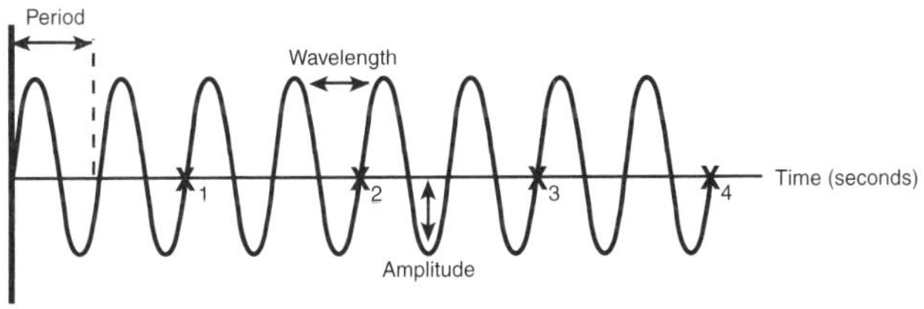

frequency = 8 cycles ÷ 4 seconds = 2 Hz

FIG. 4-1. Diagrammatic representation of a sound wave.

ultrasound pulse is transmitted by the transducer, an echo returns and appears as a spot on the trajectory of the emitted pulse. The shade of gray of the ultrasound spot is determined by the strength of the returning echo: the stronger the reflected echo pulse, the brighter the spot. By displaying images as a series of frames seen in rapid sequence, an impression of constant motion, or "**real-time**" imaging, is provided.

❍ Indications

- To guide thoracentesis, pleural biopsy, or chest tube placement. This is useful when lobar consolidation, atelectasis, pleural scarring, elevated hemidiaphragm, or loculations (such as in suspected empyema or after surgery) impair radiographic localization of free-flowing or loculated pleural fluid.
- To examine static and dynamic pleuropulmonary relationships (paradoxical movement of the diaphragm, localization of chest wall or pleural-based masses).
- To guide percutaneous needle aspiration or biopsy of pleural-based nodules and masses.

● Contraindications

- Ultrasound should not be performed over open wounds and cannot penetrate through bandages or dressings.
- Procedures may be painful over areas covered by a rash of herpes zoster, or on skin damaged by thermal or chemical injury.

❖ Equipment

Ultrasound machines should have B-mode, gray scale, real-time, and, preferably, color Doppler capabilities. Units should be easily portable to the bedside or the intensive care unit. The mechanical transducer should have a small footprint that fits easily between narrow intercostal spaces. Hardcopy images and video records are maintained for medical records, teaching, and quality control. Certain transducers with central needle guides can be purchased, but these are costly and are usually not necessary if attention is paid to fluid localization and patient positioning.

◆ Techniques

Before

The patient is seated with arms raised and resting on a table. If an invasive procedure such as thoracentesis is intended, informed consent is obtained. Ultrasound can also be performed with patients in the supine or lateral decubitus positions.

When patients are intubated and on mechanical ventilation, the head of the bed is raised to approximately 60 degrees and a rolled sheet is placed lengthwise behind the patient. While an assistant firmly grasps each end of the sheet in front of the patient, the head of the bed is lowered. The held sheet keeps the patient in a seated position, providing access to the posterior chest.

During

After applying an ample amount of gel, the transducer is moved over the posterior and lateral chest wall using real-time imaging. Ideally, the diaphragm, liver, and spleen are initially located. Then pleural fluid, loculations, and lung are visualized. Appearances most suggestive of pleural fluid include a well-defined single anechoic homogeneic space above the diaphragm (Fig. 4-2); internal divisions by septae; flapping or swirling movements made by intrapleural debris, septae, and lung; or a

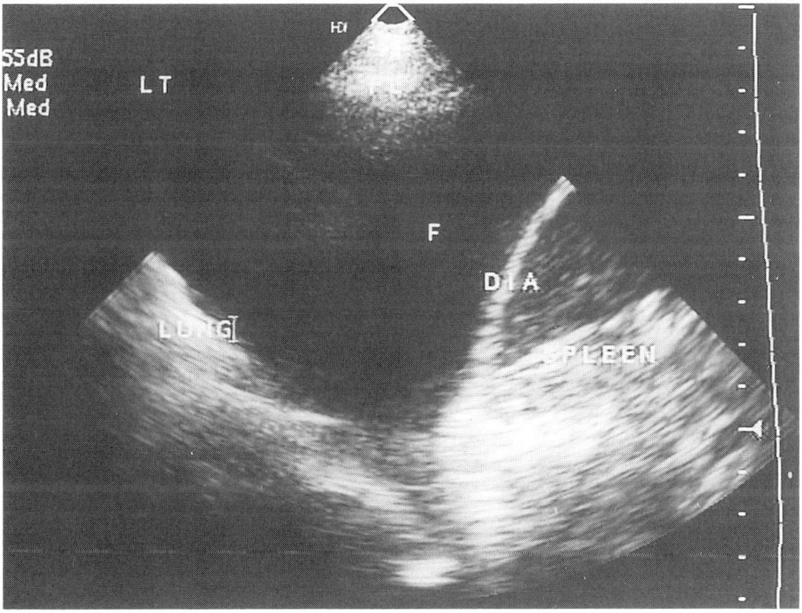

FIG. 4-2. Pleural ultrasonography demonstrating free-flowing fluid as evidenced by anechoic space (F). The diaphragm (DIA), spleen, and partially collapsed lung bathing in the fluid are readily visible.

heterogeneous space with multiple loculated areas or echogenic microbubbles (Fig. 4-3). Pleural effusions may also appear as homogeneous or heterogeneous echogenic collections (Fig. 4-4). Normal aerated lung is very echogenic, whereas consolidated lung may contain anechoic tubular structures (fluid bronchograms) or bright echogenic structures (air bronchograms).

After visualizing the diaphragm and subphrenic regions, pleural fluid is localized. If interpretation is uncertain, color Doppler should be used to differentiate fluid from solid structures such as lung or thickened pleura.

After

All of the gel is wiped off and the intercostal space through which the most pleural fluid was seen is marked in preparation for thoracentesis.

The ideal pleural ultrasonography note should contain (1) the indication for the procedure; (2) the patient's position (supine, seated, lateral decubitus); (3) a description of pleural abnormalities (approximate amount of fluid, homogeneic or heterogeneic appearance, presence of loculations or septa); (4) an estimate of chest wall or parietal pleural thickness.

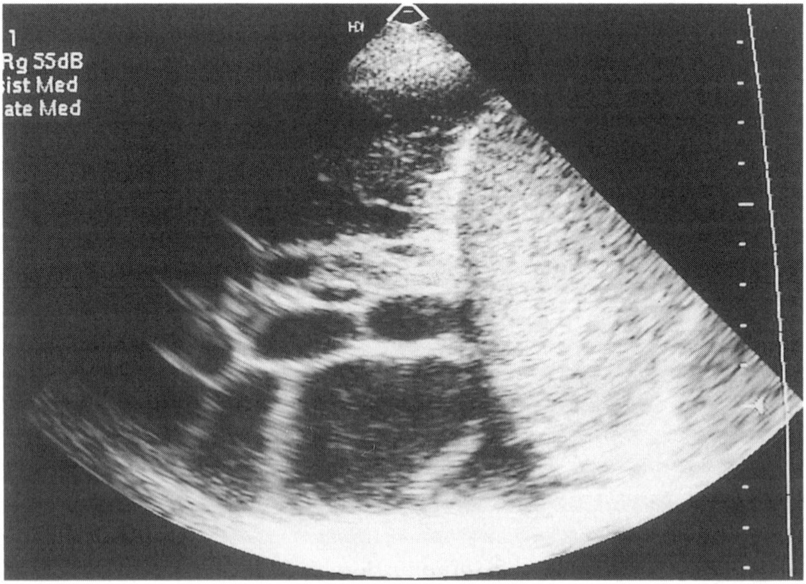

FIG. 4-3. Multiple loculations are visible in this heterogeneous appearance of a complicated parapneumonic pleural effusion.

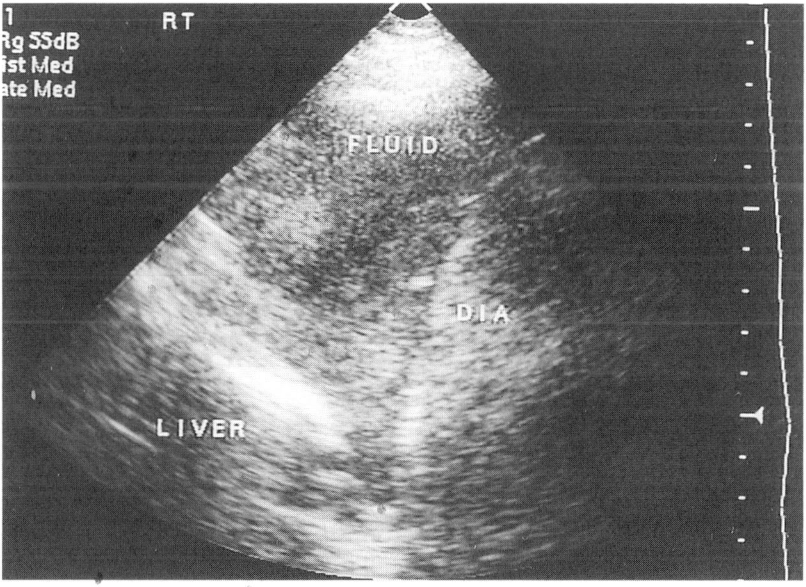

FIG. 4-4. Heterogeneous echogenic appearance of a malignant, serosanguinous pleural effusion in a patient with metastatic breast cancer.

▼ Complications

- Unsatisfactory imaging indicates that additional gel is needed or that the gain of the transducer might have to be changed.
- If substantial heterogeneity is noted, or if the space is only minimally anechoic, exploratory thoracentesis can still be attempted using a small-bore needle if the potential benefits of the procedure outweigh the potential risks of iatrogenic pneumothorax (such as in the diagnosis of complicated parapneumonic effusions, empyema, or hemothorax).

☆ Clinical Pearls

- Frequency (Hz) and maximum imaging depth (mm) are inversely related. The higher the frequency, the less the penetration depth, whereas attenuation and frequency are directly related (higher frequencies attenuate more).
- Pleural ultrasonography should be performed immediately prior to pleural procedures, without changing the patient's position or moving the patient in any way,

particularly if a very small, loculated fluid collection is noted.

- Gray scale sections facilitate the reader's ability to distinguish boundaries and discern tissue textures. Strong reflections are white. Weak echoes, such as those reflected from most pleural effusions, are dark gray.
- The information provided by pleural ultrasonography depends on the interpretative skills and experience of the ultrasonographer.

Heard on the Wards

Question: What are the advantages of pleural ultrasonography?

Answer: Pleural ultrasonography has the following advantages: (1) It provides real-time visualization of anatomic structures using nonionizing energy. (2) It can record on video and provide still photographs of pathologic processes. (3) It enhances dynamic images using color Doppler flow to detect moving fluid. (4) It is capable of diagnosing subphrenic abnormalities such as abscesses or masses. (5) It is inexpensive compared to other imaging modalities such as computed tomography. (6) It has high portability and ease of use at the bedside, particularly in critically ill patients. (7) It provides an opportunity to increase one's understanding of pleuropulmonary relationships, as well as enhance the safety of invasive pleural procedures.

Question: What is color Doppler?

Answer: Color Doppler flow imaging is a useful adjunct to real-time gray scale pleural ultrasonography. When fluid is free-flowing, colors are superimposed on the gray scale image as Doppler shift is generated (Doppler shift is audible and results from sound bouncing off fluid or blood in the pleural space).

Question: Why is it important to determine if fluid is free-flowing or loculated?

Answer: As with real estate, what really counts is location. Is this a simple effusion or an increasingly complex pleural process that may require further imaging, chest tubes drainage, or thoracoscopy? Loculated effusions are often more difficult to manage, and may be a sign of increased inflammation, infection, scarring, and lung retraction.

Question: What if I see adhesions on pleural ultrasonography?

Answer: Adhesions may explain why an effusion cannot be totally drained or why a lung does not fully reexpand after thoracentesis. Thick and even vascularized adhesions between the lung and the chest wall should be carefully avoided during chest tube insertion or thoracoscopy to prevent bleeding or inadvertent lung perforation.

Recommended Reading

Birnholz J. Chest wall and lung surface viewing with ultrasound. Chest 1988;94:1275–1276.

Eibenberger KL, Dock WI, Ammann ME, Dorffner R, Hormann MF, Grabenwoger F. Quantification of pleural effusions: sonography versus radiography. Radiology 1994;191:681–684.

Sonographic measurements correlated significantly better with effusion volume than did radiographic measurements.

Edelman SK. Understanding ultrasound physics, 2nd ed. The Woodlands, TX: ESP Inc., 1994.

A simplified approach to ultrasound physics. This is not necessarily bedtime reading material.

Goerg C, Schwerk WB, Goerg K, Walters E. Pleural effusion: an acoustic window for sonography of pleural metastases. J Clin Ultrasound 1991;19:93–97.

A good description of different patterns of pleural carcinomatosis.

Houston JG, Fleet M, Cowan MD, McMillan NC. Comparison of ultrasound with fluoroscopy in the assessment of suspected hemidiaphragmatic movement abnormality. Clin Radiol 1995; 50:95–98.

In this comparative study of 30 patients, authors found that ultrasound can detect milder abnormalities of hemidiaphragmatic movement than fluoroscopy.

Lomas DJ, Padley SG, Flower CDR. The sonographic appearances of pleural fluid. Br J Radiol 1993;66:619–624.

Dynamic features (flapping movements of septa or atelectatic lung and swirling echoes) were seen in more than 80% of cases.

McLoud TC, Flower CDR. Imaging the pleura: sonography, CT, and MR imaging. AJR 1991;156:1145–1153.

A well-written, brief review of pleural abnormalities.

Weingart JP, Guico RR, Nemcek AA, Li YP, Chiu ST. Ultrasound findings following failed clinically directed thoracenteses. Ultrasound 1994;22:419–426.

Ultrasound works when the clinical examination doesn't.

Wu R-G, Yuan A, Liaw Y-S, et al. Image comparison of real-time gray-scale ultrasound and color Doppler ultrasound for use in diagnosis of minimal pleural effusion. Am J Respir Crit Care Med 1994;150:510–514.

More than 90% of patients with pleural fluid had a positive color signal. None of the 16 patients without an effusion had a color signal.

Yang PC, Luh KT, Chang DB, Yu CJ, Kuo SH, Wu HD. Ultrasonographic evaluation of pulmonary consolidation. Am Rev Respir Dis 1992;146:757–762.

Ultrasound can be useful in the detection of microabscesses and air bronchograms.

5. THORACIC DRAINAGE DEVICES

✤ Definition

A thoracic drainage device is connected to a large- or small-bore chest tube to allow one-way evacuation of air or fluid from the pleural cavity.

■ Basic Principles

Thoracic drainage devices have evolved considerably since first introduced in the early 20th century. The primary goal of thoracic drainage devices is to continuously remove fluid or air from the pleural cavity. This is achieved by allowing gravity drainage, or by applying negative pressure to the pleural space to enhance lung reexpansion and force evacuation of air or fluid from the pleural space. Today, the one bottle and two bottle systems are of historical interest only. In fact, almost all hospitals carry commercially available disposable thoracic drainage systems whose function is based on the three-bottle or **three-container system.**

These drainage systems include a **collection chamber** into which flows air or fluid from the pleural space (container 1); a **water seal chamber** that keeps air from entering the pleural cavity, allows evacuation of air from the pleural space, and permits monitoring of negative pressures referred from the pleural cavity (container 2); and a **suction control chamber** (container 3) that regulates the amount of negative pressure being applied to the pleural space through the system. All three chambers are interconnected. Additional features include a manual high-negative-pressure release valve, an automatic high-negative-pressure release valve, a positive-pressure release valve at +2 cm H_2O, and sampling ports to remove pleural fluid from the drainage device. Negative pressure is applied to the drainage device by way of the vacuum provided by wall suction in most hospitals. Because the amount of suction being applied to the pleural space is regulated by the suction control chamber, excess suction being applied from the wall will not be detrimental. If wall suction is unavailable, a portable suction pump such as an **Emerson pump** can be placed at the bedside instead. Another drainage device is the one-way **Heimlich valve.** The principle of this device is to allow spontaneous evacuation of air through a one-way flutter valve. In case of fluid, or if suction is desired, the Heimlich valve may be attached to a collection container.

❍ Indications

- Pleural effusions or pneumothorax requiring chest tube drainage.
- To enhance lung expansion and pleural drainage after thoracoscopy or thoracotomy.
- One-way Heimlich valves are used for patients being transported or discharged home with pneumothorax and who do not require suction.

● Contraindications

- There are no contraindications to thoracic drainage devices.
- Heimlich valves should be avoided if drainage of blood, pus, or abundant pleural fluid is suspected because the valve may stick, resulting in accumulation of positive pressure in the pleural space and subsequent tension pneumothorax.

❖ Equipment

Pleur-Evac (Deknatel-Snowden-Pencer)

These plastic containers have either wet (A7000/A8000 series) or dry (A6000 series) suction mechanisms. With the wet suction mechanism, the height of a water column determines the amount of negative pressure being applied to the pleural space. Once the vacuum source is turned on, gentle bubbling through the water column assures that the amount of suction desired is actually being applied (excess negative pressure is being evacuated through the water column and is visualized as bubbling). With the dry suction mechanism, a dial on the side of the suction control chamber allows one to set the desired level of suction. An orange float on the front of the unit can be seen to rise, confirming that the desired level has been reached. If the ball is not seen, it may be necessary to increase the level of negative pressure applied from the vacuum source. To place patients to water seal (or gravity drainage), tubing between the suction control chamber and the vacuum source must be disconnected (Fig. 5-1).

Thora-Seal III (Sherwood, Davis, and Geck)

This closed-chest drainage system made of clear polycarbonate is built using the same principles as the above-described device but has a unique feature: its replaceable collection chamber can

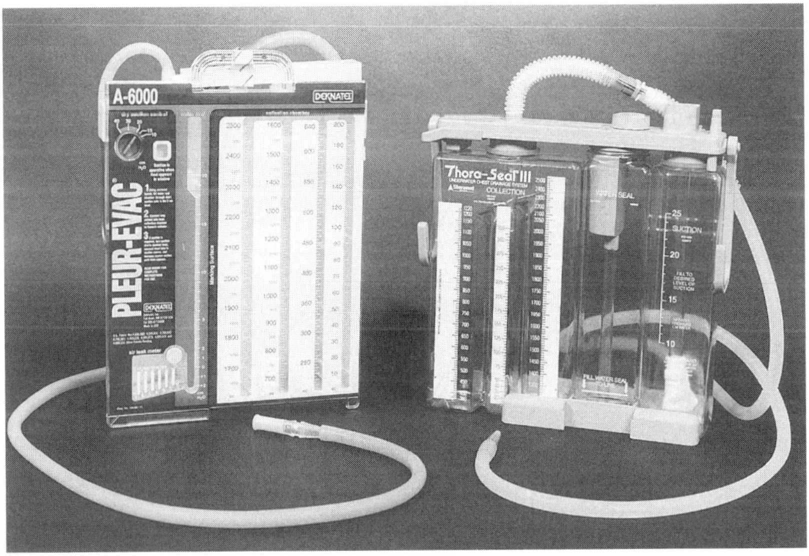

FIG. 5-1. Three-compartment chest drainage systems by Deknatel (Pleur-Evac dry suction) and Sherwood (Thora-Seal).

be removed without changing the entire chest drainage unit. Suction pressure is applied through a wet water column that can be filled to 25 cm.

The Heimlich Valve

This one-way rubber flutter valve avoids tension pneumothorax by allowing evacuation of air and excess positive intrapleural pressure during expiration, while preventing atmospheric air from entering the pleural space during inspiration. It is encased in a 15-cm-long transparent plastic tube with adapters at either extremity. These connect to the chest tube and patient. The proximal adapter can be left open to air or connected to a collection device for gravity drainage of small amounts of pleural fluid. The device is easily taped to the skin for patient transportation. Heimlich valves should be avoided if drainage of pus, blood, or abundant pleural fluid is expected. In these cases, the rubber valve may stick, making further evacuation of air or fluid impossible, and resulting in an accumulation of positive pressure within the pleural cavity (Fig. 5-2).

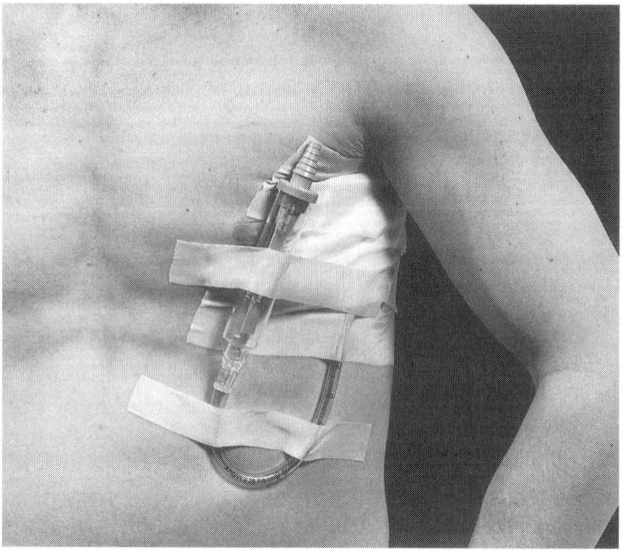

FIG. 5-2. Patient with spontaneous pneumothorax and indwelling large-bore chest tube connected to one-way Heimlich valve. The valve is positioned to avoid drainage of excess fluid from the chest during ambulation. A small square of gauze wrapped around the distal end of the valve allows both air and fluid to escape when the patient lies down.

◆ Techniques and Setting-up of Thoracic Drainage Devices

Before

The thoracic drainage device should be set up before chest tube insertion is completed. If appropriate, water is added to the suction control chamber until the desired level of negativity is reached. Water is also added to the water seal chamber, usually to the 2-cm mark.

During

The 6-foot tubing from the collection chamber is connected to the chest tube with the five-in-one connector provided, and connections are secured using a banding gun or tape. If suction is desired, the tubing from the suction control chamber is connected to the vacuum source with 6- to 10-foot-long tubing.

After

After chest tubes have been connected to the thoracic drainage device, it is necessary to (1) adjust the desired level of negative suction; (2) assure that the chest tube is functioning; (3) check for air leak (bubbling) in the water seal chamber; (4) assure that all connections between tubing are secure; (5) note the amount and type of fluid drainage into the collection chamber.

Patients who have had chest tube drainage for pneumothorax or surgery involving manipulation of visceral pleura and lung should be placed to water seal for at least several hours prior to chest tube removal. A **follow-up chest radiograph** prior to removal confirms persistent lung expansion off suction. When chest tubes are removed, the entire thoracic drainage system is discarded into a biohazard bag.

The ideal chest tube drainage surveillance note should include (1) the amount of total drainage and amount of fluid drained during the past 24 hours; (2) a description of the color of the fluid and whether there has been a change in amount or appearance; (3) the amount of negative suction being applied and whether the patient is on gravity drainage only (also frequently referred to as water seal); (4) a description of the water seal chamber and whether there is evidence of fluctuation of the water column with tidal breathing off suction; (5) a description of the water seal chamber and whether there is evidence of bubbling, signifying presence of an air leak.

▼ Complications

- Incomplete fluid drainage can occur if the suction tubing is kinked or if fluid accumulates in the loops formed by the tubing as it droops below a drainage device hung to the bed rails. Excess tubing should be coiled and laid on the bed.
- Chest tube occlusion is suggested by loss of fluctuation in the water seal chamber during tidal breathing. This occurs if the patient is lying on the tubing, or if tubing is clogged with fibrin or blood. Milking the tube by gently kneading it between two fingers can free clots and debris. Roller clamps can also be used, if available.
- Bubbling in the water seal chamber signifies an air leak between the pleural space and the water seal. This is usually from a visceral pleural tear, but can have other origins, including holes in the tubing, disconnected tubing, or breakage of the plastic drainage device itself.
- Reexpansion pulmonary edema is avoided by draining fluid gradually. When first attached in patients with pleural effusions, pleural drainage should be allowed to occur to gravity only. If more than 1,000 cm^3 of fluid is rapidly removed and no air leak is visible in the water seal chamber, the chest tube can be temporarily clamped.

- Tension pneumothorax can develop if Heimlich valves are attached backward. This is avoided by always placing the valve as directed. Each valve is embedded with an arrow and text reading either "to patient" or "to air."

☆ Clinical Pearls

- Reasons for persistent air leak in the water seal chamber include extrapleural sentinel hole, inadequate closure of the chest tube insertion site (if tight sutures are not desired, Vaseline gauze can be wrapped around the chest tube at skin level), incomplete obliteration of the subcutaneous insertion tract, a broken thoracic drainage device, holes in the connection tubing, and loose connections between chest tube and suction tubing.
- Reasons for inadequate drainage of air or fluid include insufficient levels of suction (negative pressure), kinked chest tube or suction tubing, rise of water or spillage of drainage fluid into the water seal chamber, dependent reverse loops of connection tubing, and obstruction of the chest tube by fibrin or blood clots.
- A trial of water seal drainage is probably unnecessary prior to chest tube removal in patients with chest tubes placed for pleural effusions who do not have air leaks.
- The lowest level of suction that evacuates the pleural space and maintains complete lung reexpansion is also the safest. High levels of suction in the presence of a large air leak may actually keep the visceral pleural tear open.
- When the chest tube is to water seal, and excess negative pleural pressure has been evacuated using the high negative pressure release valve, residual pleural pressure is approximately equal to the difference between the two levels of water noted in the water seal chamber.

Heard on the Wards

Question: What are the advantages of current drainage devices over the ancient three-bottle systems?

Answer: First of all, no more broken glass! Other advantages are as follows: (1) Single-use, disposable, portable units are readily available in most hospitals. (2) Once connected to the patient, few manipulations are necessary, so that the risk of bacterial contamination or accidental disconnection is small. (3) Negative pressures applied to the pleural space are easily altered, and water seal or gravity drainage is easily applied. (4) Expertise is readily acquired from practice and patient care-oriented in-services.

Question: How do I check for leaks in the system?

Answer: Leaks in the drainage system or tubing can be located by clamping the chest tube near its insertion site. If bubbling continues in the water seal chamber, the leak is somewhere between the clamp and the water seal chamber. The entire system can be examined in this manner. If, on the other hand, bubbling stops when the tube is clamped, the air leak is originating either from the pleural space or at the incision site. The chest tube dressing, therefore, should always be removed and carefully inspected. If necessary, Vaseline gauze can be wrapped around the chest tube insertion site, or additional purse-string sutures can be tied to further close the skin around the chest tube. Avoid pushing the externally contaminated chest tube back into the pleural cavity.

Question: How do I measure accurately the amount of drainage fluid when the drainage system has tipped over and fluid is in all of the columns? There are so many marking lines, and I can't read a one.

Answer: You are the "chest tube scorekeeper." You should keep a running tally on the amount of fluid drained daily. Thus, your total fluid drained is calculated by adding the amounts of fluid in each portion of the collection chamber; the amount of fluid drained in the last 24 hours is calculated by subtracting yesterday's total amount from today's calculated total.

Question: What is the role of water seal versus negative suction?

Answer: Water seal, also known as gravity drainage, allows fluid or air to flow from the pleural cavity to the chest drainage device without applying suction. The water seal chamber is the drainage device's window to the pleural space. During negative suction, higher negative pressures are being applied to the pleural space to actively aspirate air or fluid more quickly. Pressure fluctuations within the space are transmitted to the water seal chamber, usually causing a rise and fall in the water column there. Air bubbles are visible in the case of an air leak.

Question: Why does water rise in the water seal chamber every time I disconnect the chest tube from suction and place it to water seal?

Answer: This reflects the higher negative pressure left in the pleural space. This excess negativity can be vented by depressing the high negativity relief valve until the manometer shows the desired range of pleural pressure: usually 2 to 8 cm H_2O to check for fluctuation.

Question: Are there any advantages to using "dry" versus "wet" suction devices?

Answer: The dry Pleur-Evac, in addition to being quieter, will maintain constant negative pressure as long as sufficient suction is being applied from the central source (wall suction). Because there is no water column, evaporation does not occur, and negative pressure being applied will not decrease. In addition, greater levels of suction (up to –40 cm) are possible (versus a maximum of –25 for water columns).

Recommended Reading

Harris DR, Graham TR. Management of intercostal drains. Br J Hosp Med 1991;45:383–386.

Includes a summary of pitfalls and complications.

Munnell ER. Thoracic drainage. Ann Thorac Surg 1997;63: 1497–1502.

Includes a nice review of management considerations, as well as positive and negative attributes of chest tube insertion techniques.

Roe BB. Physiologic principles of drainage of the pleural space. Am J Surg 1958;96:246–253.

Although some of the information is outdated, the explanation of pleural physiology is worth reading.

Rothberg AD, Marks KH, Maisels MJ. Understanding the Pleur-Evac. Pediatrics 1981;67:482–484.

Evacuation rate is proportional to the negative pressure applied and the radius of the chest tube (Poiseuille's law).

Spouge AR, Thomas HA. Tension pneumothorax after reversal of a Heimlich valve. AJR 1992;158:763–764.

Never attach a one-way valve backward!

Symbas PN. Chest tube drainage. Surg Clin North Am 1989;69: 41–46.

Includes a simple explanation of the three-bottle system.

Teplitz L. Update: are milking and stripping chest tubes necessary? Am Assoc Clin Nurs 1991;18:506–511.

To strip or to milk? A concise description of the advantages and disadvantages of both techniques.

6. SKIN DEGERMING, DISINFECTION, AND STERILIZATION TECHNIQUES

Skin degerming is necessary in all patients undergoing invasive procedures. These procedures are readily taught on the wards, but it has been our experience that many health care providers, when questioned about products and techniques used on an almost daily basis, know little of the scientific basis surrounding such use. In addition, all invasive pleural procedures require sterile instruments. A brief overview of sterilization and disinfection procedures, therefore, is within the scope of this manual. We encourage readers, regardless of their level of expertise, to spend a few minutes with the following paragraphs, even if the content seems to be both obvious and simple at first glance.

✤ Definition

Skin **degerming** is the process by which a patient's skin is prepared before an invasive procedure. In addition to washing and degerming of the operator's hands (and wearing sterile gloves), this helps prevent procedure-related infectious complications.

Sterilization is defined as the destruction by physical or chemical processes of all life forms.

Disinfection, on the other hand, is defined as the elimination of pathogenic microorganisms other than bacterial and fungal spores from inanimate objects. High-level disinfectants can, however, be sporicidal at specific concentrations or after lengthy exposure to the organism. **Intermediate-level disinfectants** are capable of destroying vegetative bacteria, viruses, fungi, and *Mycobacterium tuberculosis,* but cannot destroy microbial spores. **Low-level disinfectants** destroy most bacteria, and some viruses and fungi, but do not destroy *M. tuberculosis* or bacterial spores.

Germicides are agents that destroy microorganisms on either living tissue or inanimate objects. Thus germicides are divided into fungicides and bactericides.

Antiseptics are agents that are capable of removing microorganisms from skin or mucous membranes by inhibition of growth or by destruction.

Decontamination is any physical or chemical process that reduces the number of microorganisms on an inanimate object sufficiently to make it safe for handling. This is usually achieved by washing with soap and water, using ultrasound cleaners, and employing automatic washers-decontaminators.

Cleaning is the simple removal of organic material. It is usually performed prior to sterilization or disinfection of medical and surgical devices.

Basic Principles

Skin Degerming Procedures

Although a variety of agents are used for skin degerming, some are more popular than others. Indeed, preferences vary in every institution. Participation in an "inservice" on skin degerming procedures can, therefore, be a beneficial experience, and helps avoid confusion or misunderstanding when performing procedures on the wards, in a procedure suite, or in the operating room.

Skin degerming is performed in order to prevent contaminating the chest wall or pleural space with bacteria residing on the skin surface. These bacteria usually are found in the epidermis, around hair follicles, sebaceous glands, and skin crevices. Bacteria that take up residence in these areas multiply readily, whereas other bacteria transiently become part of the skin flora after contamination from other sources.

Transient bacteria are readily removed by hand washing with soap or other detergents (by the way, a detergent is defined as a cleansing agent). When considering agents for skin degerming, one must consider the agent's potential for skin irritation, allergic or toxic reactions, risk of persistent activity on the skin, overall antimicrobial effect, and speed of bactericidal activity.

Sterilization Procedures

Many single-use instruments, such as chest tubes, thoracentesis kits, needles, and syringes, come in sterile prepackaged containers. However, most reusable instruments, such as trocars, stainless steel instruments, pleural biopsy needles, or even asbestos-free United States Pharmacopeia (USP)-approved talc powder, require sterilization.

Sterilization is achieved using a variety of chemical or physical agents to completely eradicate and inactivate all microorganisms, including bacterial spores. These spores are amazingly resistant to sterilization. The efficacy of the various sterilization techniques is dependent on the system being used and the microorganisms being eradicated. Most hospitals today use heat or ethylene oxide to sterilize medical and surgical devices. Sterile containers are used to store sterile equipment until use. Colored tags are usually placed on the containers to indicate sterility. If instruments are heat-sensitive or likely to be destroyed by gas sterilization, liquid chemical sterilants can be used.

❍ Indications

- Skin degerming is performed prior to every invasive diagnostic or therapeutic procedure.
- Sterilization of instruments is mandatory prior to using any instrument to invade the pleural space.

● Contraindications

There are no contraindications to skin degerming. Patients should be questioned, however, about previous reactions to agents such as iodine or topical antiseptics that may cause contact dermatitis.

❖ Equipment and Techniques

Techniques of Skin Degerming

Although skin degerming techniques may vary, all agree that it should always be performed. Before the procedure the operator should wash both hands with a povidone-iodine (Betadine) or a chlorhexidine solution for at least 2 minutes. Rinse thoroughly. Ideally, the hands should be dried with a sterile towel before gloving up with sterile gloves. The skin at the site of the procedure and the area surrounding it should be scrubbed with a povidone-iodine surgical scrub or another agent (see below) using a sponge or gauze swab. Scrubbing is done in a circular motion moving in an ever growing circle from the procedure site outward. It is usually unnecessary to cover the same area repeatedly. If the scrub was performed by an operator wearing sterile gloves, these gloves may be changed for the procedure.

Agents Used for Skin Degerming and Surgical Scrub

Isopropyl alcohol is a rapidly bactericidal water-soluble compound that acts through protein denaturation. At concentrations greater than 70%, alcohol is highly active against gram-negative bacteria, fungi, *M. tuberculosis,* and most viruses (including human immunodeficiency virus, or HIV). Because it cannot inactivate bacterial spores or hydrophilic viruses such as echovirus, it is not considered a high-level disinfectant. Alcohol readily inactivates tap water contaminants after hand washing but is often irritating to the skin after repeated use.

Hydrogen peroxide (H_2O_2) is a low-level disinfectant that, at 6% concentration, is active against most bacteria, viruses, and fungi. Its chemical cousin, **paracetic acid** (Steris), which has a broader antimicrobial activity, is often used in automated sterilization procedures of endoscopic instruments.

Chlorhexidine gluconate (Hibiclens) is a sudsing detergent that is rapidly active against most gram-positive and gram-negative bacteria. Combined with alcohol it is an effective antiseptic, and it has a cumulative antibacterial effect due to its persistence on the skin surface. It is frequently employed instead of iodine preparations in persons with reactions to iodine. Because it is minimally absorbed, is rarely irritating, and has excellent antimicrobial activity, chlorhexidine gluconate appears to be the ideal agent for skin degerming and surgical scrub for all areas except the head.

Hexachlorophene (pHisohex) is a similar sudsing agent but is not bactericidal on contact. Although bacteriostatic, it has little activity on gram-negative bacteria and is therefore not recommended as a surgical scrub.

Iodophores such as povidone-iodine are probably the most frequently used skin degerming agent. Povidone, or polyvinylpyrrolidone, is a synthetic polymer that binds iodine. Iodine is rapidly germicidal against most fungi, bacteria, spores, and viruses. Povidone-iodine is an iodophore that is as potent as iodine alone but longer acting, water-soluble, and less toxic. The higher the percentage aqueous solution, the higher the content of iodine. Iodine can cause skin irritation, rash, or burning. Patients should be asked if they have had adverse effects from iodine exposure, and if so, this should become part of their medical history. Iodophores are active against most bacteria, viruses, fungi, and *M. tuberculosis.* Because iodophores are not sporicidal they are not considered high-level disinfectants.

Techniques of High-Level Disinfection

High-level disinfection can be used for **instruments** employed in invasive procedures. This term, however, should not be confused with sterilization. Although high-level disinfectants may destroy microorganisms, they will usually not cause sterilization, which implies destruction of all microorganisms as well as bacterial spores.

High-level disinfection is usually sufficient if instruments are in contact with the skin or mucous membranes only, whereas sterilization is necessary if body cavities or viscera are involved. High-level disinfection is usually achieved, however, with a variety of sporicidal chemical agents. After thorough cleaning, instruments are placed in a bath containing the disinfectant, run through a time cycle specific to the agent employed, and ultimately rinsed and dried prior to use.

Agents Used for High-Level Disinfection

Two percent glutaraldehyde (Cidex) is a commonly used agent that eradicates most microorganisms and 99.8% of mycobacteria after 10 minutes of exposure. Most species of mycobacteria are completely inactivated after at least 20 minutes of exposure. One percent gluteraldehyde is the minimum accepted level concentration for high-level disinfection. Although this product is probably satisfactory for instruments such as flexible or rigid bronchoscopes, it is generally considered to be unsuitable for instruments used in the pleural space.

Formaldehyde (the liquid form of which is formalin) is less effective than glutaraldehyde and has many adverse effects that have led the Occupational Safety and Health Administration (OSHA) to implement specific regulations for monitoring its use. For these reasons it is no longer used as a disinfectant in health care facilities.

Techniques Used for Sterilization

Steam sterilization is the safest and probably the least expensive method of sterilization available. It is based on the use of a steam sterilizer that ensures that liquid water is heated until evaporation occurs (steam). The heat given off from steam, as well as the ability for steam to penetrate articulated surfaces and other materials, makes it an ideal sterilant. The pressure chamber used for steam sterilization is called an autoclave. Because not all microorganisms die at the same time, the duration of the sterilization cycle, as well as the amount of chamber pressure and utilization of moisture or dry heat, affects the sterilization process. Most sterilization duty cycles require at least 30 minutes of exposure at 250°F to 270°F (121°C to 132°C).

Flash sterilization is a procedure used in many operating rooms through which instruments emergently required or those inadvertently dropped on the floor during an intervention are rapidly heat-sterilized and made available for almost instant use. Flash sterilization uses steam at 132°C for 3 minutes.

Ethylene oxide sterilization, also known as EO gas sterilization, is widely used, particularly for medical and surgical products made of plastic, rubber, silk, electronic equipment, and endoscopic instruments that cannot withstand the heat and moisture of steam sterilization. EO is a colorless gas with substantial alkylating properties that cause it to interfere with the life sustaining function of DNA at the cellular level. The efficacy of EO sterilization is a function of the concentration of gas used, temperature, humidity, and exposure time. Its major disadvantage is that at least 8 to 16 hours of sterilization and aeration is required, making EO unsuitable for instruments requiring rapid turnover.

Paracetic acid is increasingly used in many hospitals. This system uses a liquid to process endoscopes and other reusable, immersible surgical devices. Sterilization time is approximately 30 minutes. Following a 10- to 12-minute exposure to the sterilant (paracetic acid) at 56°C, multiple water rinses are performed to remove sterilant residue.

▼ Complications

- Antiseptics and disinfectants can cause contact dermatitis and allergic reactions. An allergy history should always be obtained before any invasive procedure is carried out.
- Chemical sterilants cause major irritation in case of inadvertent spillage or splashing onto mucous membranes and skin. Gloves should be used when handling these agents, and all personnel should be instructed on emergency measures.
- Instruments being removed from an autoclave are hot and may cause skin burns. They should be handled carefully.
- Heat sterilization can irreversibly destroy plastic trocars, catheters, and flexible endoscopes.
- Ethylene oxide gas has been declared by OSHA as a carcinogenic, mutagenic, neurologic, and sensitization agent. Safety precautions and monitoring of employee exposure are mandatory.
- Ethylene oxide sterilization may cause fogging of endoscopic telescopes, reducing their life spans.

☆ Clinical Pearls

- Never launder lab coats or other clothing stained with Hibiclens. A permanent stain appears when the chlorhexidine gluconate mixes with chlorinated laundry cleaners' products (this actually happened to one of our trainees). For laundering, only nonchlorinated products should be used (a hint from the warning label on the Hibiclens bottle).
- Wash off all disinfectants after the procedure. Patients will thank you, clothing will not be soiled, and itching will be avoided.
- Always read the labels of any products being used. There is a lot of interesting information out there, and your awareness of it might help avoid a telephone call to your hospital infection control unit or regional poison center.
- Handwashing before *and* after every procedure (as well as after going to the restroom) is warranted.

Heard on the Wards

Question: How do I avoid embarrassing myself during a surgical scrub?

Answer: To avoid embarrassment and being labeled a novice, be sure to remove your rings or bracelets prior to washing (don't drop that wedding band in the sink, though). Also, remove the beeper attached to your waist and hand it to an assistant who can answer your pages in case you are called during the procedure.

Question: How long should I scrub before a thoracoscopy?

Answer: The length of a surgical scrub of both the operator's hands, as well as of the patient's skin, has been a focus of debate for many years. Although many questions remain unanswered, most agree that the majority of microorganisms are destroyed during the first few minutes of scrubbing and that friction caused by a gauze or sponge may be partially responsible for removal of bacteria. A single pass of antiseptic solution on the patient's skin is usually sufficient. Always wash your hands before gloving up for a procedure. If you are assisting or performing a thoracoscopy, a 5-minute scrub before donning a sterile gown and gloves is usually satisfactory.

Question: Why are there expiration dates on sterile packaging?

Answer: Because it is a Food and Drug Administration requirement.

Recommended Reading

Centers for Disease Control. Symptoms of irritation associated with exposure to glutaraldehyde–Colorado. MMWR 1987;36:190–191.

Nine of eleven nurses using glutaraldehyde developed allergic symptoms such as eye, skin, or throat irritation, nasal discomfort, chest tightness, and cough.

Crow S. Peracetic acid sterilization: a timely development for a busy healthcare industry. Infect Control Hosp Epidemiol 1992;13:111–113.

A technical description.

Martin MA, Wenzel RP. Sterilization, disinfection, and disposal of infectious waste. In: Mandell GL, Douglas RG Jr, Bennet JE, eds. Principles and practice of infectious diseases, 4th ed. New York: Churchill Livingstone, 1995.

A concisely written chapter from one of the bibles of infectious diseases.

OSHA. Occupational exposure to formaldehyde. Fed Reg (2333): 46168–46312, Code of Federal Regulations, Title 29, Part 1910, Washington, DC: OSHA, 1987.

Describes the requirements for institutions using formaldehyde solutions.

Reichert M, Young JH. Sterilization technology for the health care facility. Gaithersburg, MD: Aspen Publishers, 1997.

A carefully prepared text with 31 chapters that should serve as a reference source for every invasive procedure unit.

Rutala WA. APIC guidelines for selection and use of disinfectants. Am J Infect Control 1990;18:99–117.

An updated guideline from the Association for Practitioners in Infection Control. Designed to assist practitioners in their selection of disinfectants.

7. PHARMACOLOGIC AGENTS

Patients with pleural diseases require a wide variety of pharmacologic agents for topical antisepsis, local anesthesia, anxiolysis and sedation, analgesia, and depression. The purpose of this chapter is to describe basic pharmacologic properties of commonly used agents in order to provide the reader with a foundation for understanding the benefits and pitfalls of these medications.

Topical Antimicrobial Ointments

Basic Principles

Topical antimicrobials are rarely needed in patients undergoing pleural procedures but can be considered in patients with poorly healing chest tube or skin incision sites. These agents have variable antimicrobial activity despite good penetration through the epidermis and systemic absorption.

Indications

Topical antiseptic ointments are employed on clean or poorly healed surgical wounds to prevent further infection, control inflammation, and avoid progression to necrosis and dehiscence.

Routine use has been historically advocated to prevent infection of otherwise clean surgical wounds. Their effectiveness in this regard is unfounded.

Local application during dressing changes may be warranted if there is evidence focal of erythema and inflammation. Topical antimicrobials can be administered instead of oral antibiotics, although their effectiveness has not been well demonstrated.

Evidence of wound dehiscence should prompt a careful inspection to ascertain whether the cause for dehiscence is technical (sutures removed too soon) or infectious (evidence of inflammation, erythema, and purulent material). Topical antiseptics are frequently applied around the wound edges, but careful debridement of the wound followed by saline irrigation is probably most helpful to promote healing. Packing with dry, wet, or iodinated gauze will prevent accumulation of serous material that could serve as a nidus for infection.

Contraindications

There are no contraindications for using topical antimicrobial ointments. However, their efficacy in most circumstances has not been demonstrated convincingly.

Adverse Effects
Adverse effects include contact dermatitis, as well as hypersensitivity reactions from cutaneous exposure and systemic absorption.

Principle Topical Antimicrobial Ointments
Bacitracin is a polypeptide antibiotic primarily active against gram-positive organisms such as staphylococci and streptococci. For topical use, it is often formulated with polymyxin B or neomycin. Anaphylaxis has been rarely reported after applications onto open wounds.

Neomycin is an aminoglycoside antibiotic seldom used in topical applications today because of noted increased bacterial resistance, widely reported contact sensitivity, and possible systemic toxicity.

Polymyxin B is bactericidal against gram-negative organisms. Bacterial resistance has been rarely reported, and contact dermatitis is rare.

Mupirocin is bactericidal against *Streptococcus* (except *Enterococcus*) and *Staphylococcus aureus,* including methicillin-resistant strains. This ointment-based drug acts mostly at the skin surface and has been shown to be highly effective for the treatment of secondarily infected eczema, burns, lacerations, and leg ulcers. Although itching has been reported, contact dermatitis is rare.

Local Anesthetics

Basic Principles
Defined as a loss of sensation in a circumscribed area of the body, local anesthesia is caused by inhibition of excitation at nerve endings or blockage of conduction through peripheral nerve fibers. Local anesthetics can be used for topical anesthesia of the skin or mucous membranes, subcutaneous injection and anesthesia of deeper tissues, nerve blocks, and regional anesthesia.

The primary factors that affect local anesthetic activity are dose, injection site, and whether a vasoconstrictor is added to the preparation.

- **Dosage** is affected by altering the volume or concentration of local anesthetic injected. In practice, the greater the volume (usually expressed in milliliters) or concentration (usually expressed in percent), the greater the dose administered.
- **Site of injection** affects rapidity of onset and duration of anesthesia. For example, subcutaneous injection results in very rapid onset but short duration of anesthesia, whereas

anesthesia from an intercostal nerve block may last longer but has a slower onset of action.

- **Vasoconstrictors** such as epinephrine can be added to local anesthetics in order to decrease the rate of vascular absorption. This usually results in longer duration of anesthesia.

Indications

To prevent local and regional pain resulting from an invasive procedure.

Contraindications

Although there are no true contraindications to local infiltration anesthesia, only the smallest possible dose should be used to obtain effective anesthesia in any patient who reports a history of allergic or hypersensitivity reactions. Preparations with additives should be avoided in these individuals, and, if necessary, an agent from a different class than the offending agent can be tried.

Epinephrine should be avoided in any patient with a history of hyperthyroidism or cardiac disease. Overall, the addition of epinephrine is usually unnecessary for most pleural procedures except perhaps thoracoscopy using local anesthesia only.

Adverse Effects

Drug toxicity is related to the amount of anesthetic administered and to the drug's direct pharmacologic activity. Adverse effects include the following:

- **Central nervous system toxicity** such as drowsiness, light-headedness, nausea, shivering, muscle twitching, tremors of the facial muscles and extremities, disorientation or confusion, and even convulsions. Seizures are usually self-limited, although diazepam 5 to 10 mg by intravenous or intramuscular injection (approximately 0.1 mg/kg) can be administered.
- **Cardiovascular toxicity** such as myocardial depression and ventricular arrhythmias. Hypotension is a common complication caused by sympathetic blockade after regional (epidural) anesthesia. Treatment includes intravenous fluids, vasopressors, and, if necessary, cardiorespiratory support.
- **Hypotension**, bradycardia, peripheral vasodilation, and cardiac arrest, which can occur after rapid intravenous injection of a large dose of local anesthetic. Intravenous fluids, vasopressors, and cardiorespiratory support may be warranted.

- **Hypersensitivity reactions**, bronchospasm, angioedema, and anaphylactic shock, seen more frequently with ester-linked agents than with amide-linked agents. These complications are believed to be related to preservatives such as methylparaben used in multidose vials. Bronchospasm should be treated with an inhaled bronchodilator such as albuterol. In case of **anaphylactic shock**, epinephrine 0.5 mL (1:1,000 solution) in 10 mL of saline should be administered intravenously and repeated every 5 minutes as necessary. Intubation and ventilatory support may be warranted. Antihistamines (hydroxyzine 50 mg by intravenous injection) and corticosteroids (Solu-Medrol 125 mg intravenous injection) are often added, but should not be expected to have an immediate effect.

Principle Local Anesthetic Agents

Lidocaine hydrochloride (Xylocaine) is the most commonly used aminoamide agent for infiltration anesthesia. Its onset of action is almost immediate. It can be used in 1%, 2%, and 4% concentrations. The addition of epinephrine prolongs the duration of action. A dose of 300 mg (15 mL of 2% solution, or 30 mL of 1% solution) is usually sufficient for most pleural procedures. The maximal single dose is 500 mg (25 mL of 2% solution). Lidocaine is longer lasting, more potent, and has a faster onset of action than its ester-linked counterpart, procaine, at similar concentrations. However, it is twice as toxic if inadvertently administered intravascularly.

Mepivacaine (Carbocaine Hydrochloride) is an aminoamide agent similar to lidocaine in terms of potency and toxicity, but has a longer duration of action because it has lesser vasodilator activity. Like lidocaine, the maximal single dose is 7 mg/kg.

Bupivacaine (Marcaine) is an aminoamide agent that is about four times as potent as lidocaine. It has a significantly longer duration of action (several hours). For these reasons, and because sensory anesthesia can be obtained without motor blockade, this agent is frequently used for major nerve blocks and epidural analgesia. Potential toxicity, however, is greater than that of lidocaine. For infiltration anesthesia, the maximal single dose should not exceed 200 mg in 24 hours (80 mL of a 0.25% solution). Bupivacaine (20 mL of 0.25% solution) provides long-lasting analgesia after infiltration around chest tube incision sites.

Cocaine is perhaps the most (in)famous of ester-linked local anesthetics. This agent has excellent topical anesthetic properties and causes significant vasoconstriction. For these reasons, it was historically used to constrict nasal mucosa prior to flexible bronchoscopy or nasotracheal intubation. Its potential for systemic toxicity and risk of addiction make it unsuitable for general use today.

Procaine Hydrochloride (Novocaine) was the first local anesthetic used for infiltration anesthesia. Because this ester-linked agent has a slower onset of action, lesser duration of anesthesia, and increased toxicity (allergic reactions including anaphylaxis after repeated use are related to rapid hydrolysis of procaine to para-aminobenzoic acid), it has been replaced by lidocaine. The maximal single dose should not exceed 14 mg/kg.

Tetracaine (Pontocaine) is an ester-linked local anesthetic at least ten times more potent than procaine, but also significantly more toxic, particularly when larger doses are used. Its toxicity and slow onset of action have led to its general abandonment for all but spinal anesthesia. Because of its long duration of action, some advocate its use for topical anesthesia of patients undergoing flexible bronchoscopy.

Anxiolytics, Hypnotics, and Sedatives

Basic Principles

The major anxiolytics belong to the benzodiazepine family. Effects are mediated through gamma-aminobutyric acid (GABA). Medication is well absorbed from the gastrointestinal tract. The onset of action of most agents is slow and erratic after intramuscular injection (5 to 15 minutes) with an average duration of action of approximately 2 hours. Onset of action after intravenous injection, however, is rapid (less than 5 minutes) with an average duration of 15 to 60 minutes.

Indications

These medications are used prior to and during invasive pleural procedures to reduce procedure-related anxiety, promote sleep, and cause anterograde amnesia.

Premedication is warranted if patients manifest a desire for medication or if apprehension persists despite a carefully obtained informed consent. It is probably unfair to assume that physicians and nurses are able to reliably assess whether patients are anxious.

Contraindications

These agents should be avoided in patients with known or suspected allergic or idiosyncratic reaction, and acute narrow-angle glaucoma (which is a contraindication for most benzodiazepines).

Patients with respiratory insufficiency or obstructive sleep apnea are at increased risk of respiratory failure. Agents should be used with caution, and only if pulmonary resuscitative equipment is available.

Adverse Effects

Adverse effects include, but are not limited to, allergic and idiosyncratic reactions such as bronchospasm, urticaria, pruritus, hypotension, and anaphylactic shock as well as respiratory depression, hypoxemia, and hypercapnia.

Relaxation of hypopharyngeal and laryngeal muscles facilitates aspiration and upper airway obstruction.

Risks for excessive sedation, confusion, drowsiness, and anterograde amnesia (often a desired effect) are at times counterbalanced by risks of disinhibition accompanied by increased agitation and combativity.

Principle Anxiolytics and Sedatives

Diazepam (Valium) is a benzodiazepine that is erratically absorbed after intramuscular injection. Its high lipid solubility causes it to enter the brain quickly. Its mechanism of action is primarily through increased inhibitory effect of GABA. In addition, diazepam raises the threshold of toxicity of local anesthetics and produces some amnesia. Like all benzodiazepines, sedation can be accompanied by impaired psychomotor function and respiratory insufficiency. Dosage is usually 2 to 20 mg by intravenous or intramuscular injection.

Lorazepam (Ativan) is a benzodiazepine with a shorter elimination half-life and good anterograde amnesic effect. Duration of action after a single dose is 12 to 24 hours. Dosage is usually 40 μg/kg by intravenous injection or 1 to 2 mg by oral route.

Midazolam (Versed) is another increasingly used benzodiazepine. Dosage is usually 1 to 10 mg by intravenous injection. Midazolam administration can result in disinhibition and agitation, but usually produces drowsiness and appears to have an excellent anterograde amnesic effect. Its half-life is the least of all the benzodiazepines currently available.

Flurazepam (Dalmane) is a benzodiazepine administered orally at bedtime (usual dose 15 to 30 mg). Abrupt discontinuation can precipitate withdrawal symptoms.

Flumazenil (Romazicon) is a benzodiazepine antagonist that can be used in case of overdose with benzodiazepines. Initial dose is 0.2 mg administered by rapid (15 to 30 seconds) intravenous injection. The dose can be repeated at 1-minute intervals for up to 4 minutes. The effects of this agent (particularly for reversal of respiratory insufficiency) subside prior to the effects of benzodiazepines, so prolonged observation is necessary until patients are fully awake.

Hydroxyzine (Vistaril) is the only nonneuroleptic antihistamine with analgesic properties and is therefore preferable to other antihistamines such as diphenhydramine (Benadryl). **Antihistamines** can be used alone or, more frequently, in addition to other pharmaceutical agents as part of a premedication regimen formulated to improve patient tolerance, comfort, and cooperation during invasive pleural procedures. Metabolized in the liver, hydroxyzine has antiemetic, anxiolytic, and antimuscarinic (bronchodilatory, antiarrhythmic, and antisialogogic) properties. It causes sedation and increases the effects of opioid analgesics and other central nervous system depressants. A potential side effect is excessive drowsiness, which may require observation and supportive care in case of respiratory insufficiency. Dosage is 25 to 100 mg by intramuscular injection. Hydroxyzine in combination with an intramuscular injection of morphine will provide analgesia for 2 to 6 hours.

Analgesics

Basic Principles

Analgesics are used to prevent or treat nociceptive and neuropathic pain related to an invasive procedure or due to the effects of an underlying illness. Effect is usually a function of the pharmacologic properties of the agent used, dose, and mode of administration. The benefits of effective pain control must be weighed against a medication's side effects. This balancing act should be carefully explained to patients and their caregivers. Often, several agents must be tried before an effective and satisfactory balance is finally achieved.

Pain is defined as an unpleasant sensory and emotional experience associated with actual or potential tissue damage. Noxious stimuli are transmitted from sensory nerve endings along neural pathways to the spinal cord and brain (primarily the brainstem and thalamus). These stimuli are then modulated, probably at the periaqueductal gray matter (midbrain) and rostroventral medulla. The dorsal horn, however, seems to be the gateway of nociception. Thus, specific pharmacologic agents can control the transmission and modulation of painful stimuli through the manipulation of neurotransmitters (such as serotonin and epinephrine). This is known as the **gate control** theory of analgesia.

It is well recognized that pain is usually inadequately managed. Reasons for this include cultural differences in patients' response and tolerance to pain, wide variability of patients' response to different analgesics, the overall subjective nature of the pain response itself, and underlying difficulties in measuring pain and the effects of analgesics.

Pain from pleural diseases is often unrelenting, inhibits breathing, and is often accompanied by high-grade anxiety or depression. It is easily demoralizing for patients and their families, interferes with sleep and nutrition, and prohibits patients from thinking clearly. The simple fear of pain will often interfere with an individual's making reasonable choices about diagnostic and therapeutic alternatives, lifestyle, or end-of-life issues. In most cases, patients will consider pain to be an emergency. Think about it.

Indications

Analgesics are warranted to decrease a patient's perception of pain caused by a procedure. Analgesics are also necessary to treat pain and discomfort related to a patient's underlying illness, such as pleuritic pain from effusion or infection, or pain radiating from tumors involving the chest wall.

Contraindications

There are no contraindications to pain control, although specific precautions are warranted when using certain agents.

Adverse Effects

Adverse effects at the level of the central nervous system, cardiorespiratory system, hepatorenal system, and gastrointestinal system are dependent on the pharmacology of each analgesic agent. Deleterious effects also vary depending on the patient's underlying clinical status (e.g., presence of breathing difficulties, kidney or liver failure, or impaired mental status).

Tolerance (defined as decreased effect of a drug after repeated administration) may, in part, be related to the wide variability of individuals' responses to different pharmacologic agents. When tolerance is suspected, and increased amounts of analgesics are required, consultation from a pain specialist is desirable. However, fear of tolerance, dependence, and untoward effects from medication frequently prompt physicians to undertreat, rather than overtreat, patients with pain.

Principle Analgesic Agents

Acetaminophen (Tylenol) is a paracetaminophol derivative with analgesic and antipyretic properties, but without antiinflammatory effects. Its mechanism of action is unknown. Peak concentrations after oral ingestion are usually reached within an hour.

Most acute procedure-related pain, such as that associated with closed-needle pleural biopsy or chest tube removal, can be treated with less than 4 g of acetaminophen daily.

Metabolized by the liver and excreted by the kidney, its major **adverse effect** is liver toxicity. Decreased dosage in patients with liver cirrhosis is warranted. Large (10 to 15 g) doses or chronic acetaminophen use can result in hepatic necrosis, the treatment of which is acetylcysteine. Unlike aspirin, acetaminophen has few side effects when normal dosages are used (300 to 500 mg every 4 hours), does not interfere with platelet function, and is associated with rare hypersensitivity reactions.

Nonsteroidal antiinflammatory drugs (NSAIDs) are quite effective analgesics for relieving mild or moderate pain, and also have antipyretic and antiinflammatory properties. They can be used alone or in combination with opioids and other analgesics. Regardless of the NSAID administered, a peak analgesic effect occurs after which increased dosing is only accompanied by greater antiinflammatory effects or adverse reactions. NSAIDs are rapidly absorbed from the gastrointestinal tract, although half-life varies depending on which preparation is used. If one class of NSAIDs is not effective in relieving pain, a NSAID of another class should be tried. A 2-week trial is usually recommended before switching to another agent.

In patients with benign pleural disease–related pain, such as pleurisy following trauma, open heart surgery, pulmonary embolism, parapneumonic effusions, or connective tissue and rheumatologic disorders, NSAIDs can be used alone. In patients with malignant pleural disease–related pain, such as malignant mesothelioma, NSAIDs are usually used in addition to opioids.

Adverse reactions include erosive gastritis and gastric hemorrhage, inhibition of platelet aggregation, nephrotoxicity (particularly in patients with congestive heart failure, hepatic cirrhosis, or in patients who are volume-depleted), fluid retention, hyperkalemia, exacerbations of bronchospasm, pulmonary infiltrates, asymptomatic transaminasemia, skin reactions, and aseptic meningitis. NSAIDs should not be administered if patients have a history of peptic ulcer disease or chronic alcohol use. Caution is warranted if patients are elderly or are taking anticoagulants.

Commonly used medications include salicylic acids, such as **aspirin** and **diflunisal** (Dolobid); acetic acids, such as **indomethacin** (Indocin) and **diclofenac** (Voltaren); propionic acids, such as **ibuprofen** (Motrin) and **naproxen** (Naprosyn); anthranilic acids, such as **meclofenamate** (Meclomen); pyrazoles, such as **phenylbutazone** (no longer used because of bone marrow toxicity); and oxicams, such as **piroxicam** (Feldene). These preparations are all administered orally.

Ketorolac (Toradol) is the only NSAID commercially available and approved for intravenous or intramuscular injection in the United States (although it also comes in an oral preparation). Ketorolac is a pyrole acetic acid with an analgesic effect approximately 6 times that of indomethacin and an antipyretic effect 20 times that of aspirin. Clearance is reduced in the elderly and in patients with renal disease. Peak plasma concentrations are achieved approximately 60 minutes after intramuscular injection and last for about 6 hours. Dosage is 30 mg by intramuscular injection every 6 hours after an initial loading dose of 60 mg.

Opioids (derived from the opium poppy) are endogenous or exogenous (natural or synthetic) substances with morphine-like properties. Exogenous opioids produce their analgesic effect by mimicking the effects of endogenous opioids on opiate receptors located in the brain and elsewhere in the central nervous system. It is therefore usually unnecessary to combine opioids to achieve analgesia.

The term **narcotic** is often used to describe opioids but is actually a misnomer, since narcotic means any drug that causes narcosis. Although opioids are generally classified as agonists (producing analgesia), agonist-antagonists, and antagonists, only those agonists most likely to be used in patients with pleural diseases will be described.

Morphine sulfate is the major opioid derived from the opium poppy. Wide variations may be noted between patients in regard to total body clearance, minimum analgesic concentrations (i.e., the least amount of drug necessary to produce an analgesic effect), and duration of pain relief. Because morphine is cleared from the plasma in less than 10 minutes after a bolus intravenous injection of 1 to 5 mg, it should probably not be used intravenously for acute pain relief unless concomitant continuous infusion is also provided.

- **Continuous intravenous infusion**, such as that used for patient-controlled analgesia (PCA) through a peripheral or central intravenous line, is highly effective and has predictable pharmacokinetics
- **Intramuscular** deltoid injection of morphine results in more rapid absorption than after gluteal muscle injection. Maximum plasma concentrations occur within 5 to 60

minutes. An initial dose of 5 to 10 mg by intramuscular injection will often result in a rapid analgesic effect, such as that needed during chest tube insertion.

- **Oral preparations** are warranted for patients with chronic pain. The oral bioavailability of morphine is one third that of the intravenous dose, so doses per 24 hours must be tripled when converting from intravenous to oral morphine. Elixir and suppository preparations are also available.
- **Immediate-release** oral morphine (MS-IR 15- and 30-mg tablets) has an onset of action of approximately 15 minutes and a duration of 3 to 4 hours. A **sustained-release** preparation (such as MS Contin or Roxanol-SR 30 mg PO) has a prolonged duration of action to 8 to 12 hours.

Meperidine (Demerol) is another commonly used opioid. Meperidine is less potent, has a faster onset of action, and has greater local anesthetic effects but may cause greater euphoria in patients than morphine. The atropine-like effects of meperidine, however, may cause tachycardia, and its byproducts may promote seizures. As part of a preprocedure premedication package, dosage is 25 to 100 mg by intramuscular injection. Meperidine can cause tachycardia, hypotension, and hyperthermia in patients taking monoamine oxidase (MAO) inhibitors.

Hydromorphone (Dilaudid) is a synthetic oral opioid that is rapidly absorbed from the gastrointestinal tract. It is at least 6 times more potent than morphine, and has a faster onset of action and shorter half-life. Dosage is 1 to 4 mg PO every 3 hours.

Oxycodone (Percocet and Percodan) and **hydrocodone** (Vicodin) are oral opioids with actions similar to those of morphine but are combined with acetaminophen. Dosage is 1 to 2 tablets PO daily not to exceed 8 tablets.

Codeine is a weak opioid with a rapid onset but short duration of action. Most health care providers are familiar with preparations combined with acetaminophen (Tylenol with codeine). Dosage is 1 to 2 tablets PO every 6 hours using 7.5 to 60 mg of codeine combined with 300 mg of acetaminophen. Use is often limited because of acetaminophen-related side effects. An elixir is available.

Fentanyl is currently the most frequently used intravenous intraoperative analgesic. In general, fentanyl is 100 times more potent than morphine. Its onset of action is rapid but its half-life appears to be longer than that of morphine. If used repeatedly by intravenous injection, subsequent respiratory depression may be seen.

- Its lipid-soluble relative, **alfentanil**, has a very short half-life, allowing precise monitoring of intraoperative concentrations.
- For patients with chronic pain, a **fentanyl patch** (Duragesic) can be employed. Starting dosage is usually one transdermal 25-μg patch every 3 days.

Adverse effects of opioids include respiratory depression, nausea, vomiting, constipation, urinary retention, pruritis, and physical or psychological dependence. Respiratory depression should be suspected if patients develop a decreased rate of breathing with a compensatory increased tidal volume. Severe hypoxemia and hypercapnia may occur, particularly in patients with preexisting lung disease or when high doses of opiates are used.

- Prophylactic laxatives such as Senokot 2 (two tablets PO at bedtime), Dulcolax (10 mg PO at bedtime), milk of magnesia (30 cm^3 PO), an increased fluid intake, and Metamucil (1 tablespoon every morning with prune juice) will usually relieve **constipation**.
- Metachlopromide (10 mg PO or IM) will effectively increase gastrointestinal motility and relieve **nausea**.
- An antihistamine such as diphenhydramine (Benadryl 25 to 50 mg every 6 hours) will relieve **pruritus**.
- Atropine will usually block **hypotension** and **bradycardia** that occur from arteriolar vasodilatation.
- Observation, ventilatory support, and supplemental oxygenation should be instituted in cases of **respiratory depression**. For immediate reversal, administer **naloxane hydrochloride** (Narcan): one ampoule (0.4 mg/cm^3) diluted in 10 cm^3 of normal saline solution, then injected intravenously at a dose of 1 cm^3 (0.04 mg) until the respiratory rate is greater than 8 breaths per minute.
- **Physical dependence** is due to the pharmacologic properties of the analgesic (opioids) and implies withdrawal symptoms if the drug is tapered too rapidly. A slow taper over at least 14 days is warranted to allow the body to make endogenous opioids. In case of withdrawal symptoms, the drug can be reintroduced and tapered more slowly. Unlike benzodiazepines and barbiturates, opioid withdrawal is never life threatening.
- **Psychological dependence**, also known as **addiction**, is a behavioral disorder in which compulsive drug use, drug hoarding, drug craving, and return to drug use after drug detoxification occurs. Addiction is an extremely rare occur-

rence in patients with either acute or chronic pain syndromes, and is rarely encountered other than in patients with a prior history of drug abuse. Behavior modification and referral for drug detoxification is warranted. The fear of addiction should not prevent health care providers from prescribing opioids in sufficient doses to manage pain.

Antidepressants

Basic Principles

Antidepressants have no role in the treatment of procedure-related discomfort but are mentioned here because of their potential benefit in patients with chronic cancer-related pain. Many of these individuals may actually be using antidepressants to treat disease-related depression. When used for analgesia, however, doses can be reduced. It appears that most neuropathic pain syndromes respond to antidepressants. These oral drugs are well absorbed by the gastrointestinal tract and have long half-lives.

Indications

Antidepressants are warranted to treat clinically significant depression but may also be used as coanalgesics for patients with chronic pain syndromes.

Contraindications

These drugs should be avoided in patients with narrow-angle glaucoma or during the recovery phase after myocardial infarction. Caution is warranted in patients with preexisting cardiovascular disease.

Adverse Effects

Adverse effects to antidepressants include anticholinergic effects (dry mouth, urinary retention, and constipation), antihistamine effects (drowsiness), α_1-adrenergic blockade effects (orthostatic hypotension), arrhythmias, and antidopaminergic effects (dystonia).

- If patients stop taking their drug suddenly, they may notice sleep disruption and vivid dreams.
- Whenever prescribing an antidepressant to patients with a terminal illness, such as pleural carcinomatosis or malignant mesothelioma, consideration must be given to potential suicide from drug overdose of these agents, or any drug for that matter.

Principle Antidepressant Agents

Amitriptyline, a tricyclic that inhibits serotonin and norepinephrine, is the antidepressant most frequently used for pain relief. It should not be used in patients with narrow-angle glaucoma. Dosage begins usually with 25 mg PO before bedtime (10 mg single dose in the elderly), which can be gradually increased to 100 mg.

Doxepin and **imipramine** are other tricyclics that can be started at this dose.

Nortriptyline is often recommended in the elderly because it has fewer cardiovascular side effects and can be given in a smaller dose than the other tricyclics.

☆ Clinical Pearls

- Maximal respiratory depression occurs about 7 minutes after an intravenous injection of morphine and up to 30 minutes after an intramuscular injection.
- In 1806, Friedrich Wilhelm Serterner called his active opium alkaloid morphine, after Morpheus, the Greek god of dreams.
- Brownie points are never awarded for *not* giving enough local anesthetic.
- Analgesics can usually be rapidly tapered after the first 24 to 48 hours after chest tube insertion or thoracoscopy.
- Physical or psychological dependence should only be of concern when treating patients with chronic pain from benign processes. In these instances, it is best to consult a pain specialist.
- Postthoracoscopy and postthoracotomy pain syndromes may result from intercostal nerve injury or small neuromas that form along the scar. Symptoms include intermittent burning, dysesthesias, and allodynia (pain from a stimulus that usually does not cause pain) along the scar. In patients with a history of cancer, chest wall tumor invasion should always be excluded.

Heard on the Wards

Question: Are some patients at greater risk for perioperative wound infections than others?

Answer: Risk factors for perioperative wound infection include diabetes, advanced age, severe obesity, concomitant hemodialysis, corticosteroids, malnutrition, and an active infection site remote from the operative field. These risks were noted in patients undergoing traditional open surgical procedures. It is unclear whether patients undergoing endoscopic procedures have the same risks.

Question: How can I prevent perioperative wound infections?
Answer: Perioperative wound infections, although rare after the pleural procedures described in this manual, can be largely prevented by careful washing and gloving of the operator's hands; wearing masks; using sterile drapes; careful use of skin degerming procedures; minimizing hospital stay before the procedure to avoid hospital-acquired resistant organisms; shaving hair as close to the time of the procedure as possible; and treating infections at sites remote from the operative field.

Question: Are prophylactic antibiotics warranted before thoracoscopy?
Answer: Many operators advocate using cefazolin (Ancef) 1 to 2 g IV at the time of anesthesia for patients undergoing thoracoscopy. It is unclear whether antibiotics need to be continued beyond 24 hours after the procedure.

Question: Is endocarditis prophylaxis recommended for patients undergoing pleural procedures?
Answer: No. Endocarditis prophylaxis is not recommended in case of incision or biopsy of surgically scrubbed skin. Prophylaxis is warranted (amoxicillin 2 g 1 hour before the procedure) in patients undergoing rigid bronchoscopy or surgical procedures involving the respiratory tract because of the risk of bacteremia and tracheobronchial mucosal damage. In case of allergy to penicillin, clindamycin (600 mg PO), cephalexin (2.0 g PO), or azithromycin (500 mg PO) is recommended. If the patient is unable to take oral medication, ampicillin (2.0 g IM or IV), clindamycin (600 mg IV), or cefazolin (1.0 g IM or IV) can be administered 30 minutes before the procedure.

Question: Should I routinely use topical antiseptic ointments on chest tube wounds?
Answer: Probably not. Although these agents are traditionally advocated, the efficacy of topical antiseptics for preventing infection from forming has never been proven, in part because clean wounds hardly ever become infected.

Question: How do I treat wound dehiscence of a chest tube incision site?
Answer: If there is evidence of wound dehiscence, careful inspection is warranted. Povidone-iodine is applied to the skin

surrounding the wound. Necrotic tissue is removed using sterile instruments, and the wound should be rinsed with sterile saline solution or a low- to intermediate-level disinfectant. If purulent material is present, a sterile swab specimen can be sent to the microbiology laboratory for analysis. Topical or systemic antimicrobials are administered to cover the most frequently encountered pathogens, which are *Streptococcus* and *Staphylococcus aureus*. If the patient complains of local discomfort, a nonsteroidal antiinflammatory agent such as ibuprofen is prescribed.

Question: What is the difference between nociceptive and neuropathic pain?

Answer: Nociceptive pain occurs with an uninjured nervous system (e.g., pain from needle insertion into the parietal pleura, or pain from a chest tube pressing onto the apical pleura). Neuropathic pain, which is often refractory to medication, results from injury to the nervous system (e.g., postthoracoscopy or postthoracotomy pain syndrome whereby intercostal nerves have been crushed or severed, or malignant mesothelioma with invasion of intercostal nerves).

Question: What is patient-controlled analgesia and when should I use it?

Answer: Patient-controlled analgesia (PCA) allows patients to control their own dose and frequency of analgesics by means of an external drug-dispensing device. The medication (usually morphine) is delivered intravenously, allowing patients to receive medication for pain relief while minimizing side effects such as sedation. Patients do not have to rely on nursing personnel for their dosing. Continuous infusion dose is preset on the external device, as is the time interval and amount for each bolus dose. We use PCA in hospitalized patients for at least the first 2 to 3 days after thoracoscopy (continuous infusion 1 to 4 mg per hour, bolus dose 2 mg, maximum delivery possible only every 8 minutes).

Question: How do I treat a patient with metastatic pleural disease who has been on opiates and has constipation that has not responded to simple laxatives.

Answer: This can be a very uncomfortable situation for both the patient and the caregivers. Try administering a fleet enema after stool softeners and laxatives; or, when all else fails, try magnesium citrate or Go-Lytly. Warn the patient that these are big guns requiring a nearby toilet!

Recommended Reading

Alpert CC, Baker JD, Cooke JE. A rational approach to anaesthetic premedication. Drugs 1989;37:219–228.

Dajani AS, Taubert KA, Wilson W, et al. Prevention of bacterial endocarditis: recommendations by the American Heart Association. JAMA 1997;277:1794–1799.

Updated recommendations from the American Heart Association that include major changes for individuals at risk for bacterial endocarditis, such as elimination of follow-up antibiotic doses, should be present in every procedure area.

Ferrante FM, VadeBoncouer TR. Postoperative pain management. New York: Churchill Livingstone, 1993.

A reference source that covers the complex science behind pain management.

Irving GA, Wallace MS. Pain management for the practicing physician. New York: Churchill Livingstone, 1997.

Full of algorithms and flow diagrams that are readily useful to primary care physicians managing patients with chronic pain syndromes.

Mersky H. Classification of chronic pain: description of chronic pain syndrome and definition of pain terms. Pain 1986 (Suppl 3):S1.

A "must-have" of definitions.

Patt RB. Cancer pain. Philadelphia: JB Lippincott, 1993.

A comprehensive reference for practitioners caring for patients with cancer-related pain. Describes many of the invasive procedures available for pain management.

Tunkel AR. Topical antibacterials. In: Mandell GL, Douglas RG Jr, Bennet JE, eds. Principles and practice of infectious diseases, 4th ed. New York: Churchill Livingstone, 1995.

Concise and relatively complete review in a textbook that has become part of every medical library.

8. PRIMER OF DIFFERENTIAL DIAGNOSIS OF PLEURAL DISEASES

Patients with pleural disease always present a diagnostic and therapeutic challenge. An effective way of approaching these patients is to develop a **differential diagnosis** based on clinical suspicion and review of conventional chest radiographs. The diagnosis is then refined based on interpretation of the results of thoracentesis or closed-needle pleural biopsy, additional imaging studies as needed, and clinical course. Medical thoracoscopy may be warranted for definitive diagnosis. Often, several therapeutic alternatives are available. Treatment should be individualized based on the disease process, available resources, prognosis, and the patient's desires. A **multidisciplinary team approach** involving primary care providers, chest physicians and surgeons, and interventional radiologists is often desirable.

Diagnosis of Pleural Effusions

The first step in determining the cause of a pleural effusion is to define it in terms of being **a transudate or an exudate.** Thus, any new pleural effusion, except if the patient has obvious congestive heart failure, should be sampled. **Transudates** are caused by differences in osmotic relationships, usually from renal, liver, or cardiac disease. **Exudates** are caused by pleural inflammatory processes, most frequently resulting from cancer, infection, collagen vascular disease, occupational exposures such as asbestos, pulmonary embolism, or infarction, or chronic and acute inflammatory states. Fluid usually accumulates as a result of decreased lymphatic clearance or increased capillary permeability.

Although several "new" tests (such as pleural fluid cholesterol, serum/effusion albumin ratios, and effusion/fluid bilirubin ratios) have been proposed, none differentiate transudates and exudates as well as **Light's criteria**. Exudative effusions meet at least one of the following, whereas transudates meet none: (1) pleural fluid protein divided by serum protein greater than 0.5; (2) pleural fluid lactate dehydrogenase (LDH) divided by serum LDH greater than 0.6; and (3) pleural fluid LDH greater than two thirds the upper limit of normal for serum LDH. These "modified" criteria appropriately classify 99% of effusions. Contrary to common belief, there is no such thing as a "borderline" exudate.

The **differential diagnosis** of pleural effusions is further narrowed based on fluid analyses. Of course, fluid should always be sent to microbiology and cytology. **Fluid appearance** may be suggestive of certain disease processes. Usually, normal-appearing, or **serous**, pleural fluid is straw-colored or slightly serosanguinous. **Turbid** fluid may be suggestive of infection or increased lipid content. **Viscous** fluid may be suggestive of malignant mesothelioma. Fluid with high cholesterol levels may have a characteristic satin-like sheen. **Chylous** or pseudochylous fluid may appear milky. Dark reddish brown fluid may be suggestive of old blood in the pleural space. If fluid appears **bloody**, a hematocrit greater than 50% of the peripheral blood hematocrit confirms a hemothorax. **White blood cell (WBC) counts** in pleural fluid are usually less than 5,000/mm^3; counts above 10,000/mm^3 suggest infection. **Lymphocytosis** suggests chronicity of the effusion, and more than 50% of small lymphocytes should prompt suspicions of malignancy or tuberculosis.

Pleural fluid **eosinophilia** is caused by air or blood in the pleural space. Although it has been taught that eosinophilic effusions are usually benign, recent studies suggest that malignancy occurs as frequently with eosinophilia as without. Other causes of eosinophilic effusions include parasitic diseases (hydatid cyst, ascariasis, amebiasis, or paragonimiasis), drug reactions, and Churg-Strauss syndrome. **Mesothelial cells** usually make up more than 1% of cells in pleural fluid. They are reportedly rare in effusions caused by tuberculosis, complicated parapneumonic effusions, and after pleurodesis.

Pleural fluid glucose is usually greater than 60 mg/dL and parallels serum values. If lower, the differential diagnosis includes cancer, tuberculosis, parapneumonic effusion, and rheumatoid disease. Pleural **fluid amylase** levels need not be measured routinely but should be obtained if pancreatic disease, including pseudocysts, or esophageal rupture is suspected. In these cases, levels are often higher than serum values.

Normal **pleural fluid pH** is often greater than 7.65. Patients with suspected parapneumonic effusions and pleural fluid pH levels below 7.0 are classified as having a "complicated parapneumonic effusion" that usually requires immediate drainage to avoid the morbidity of subsequent empyema. Actually, a fluid pH level less than 7.20 usually narrows the differential diagnosis to only ten disease processes. These are (1) rheumatoid arthritis; (2) esophageal perforation; (3) acidosis; (4) cancer; (5) hemothorax; (6) tuberculosis; (7) urinothorax; (8) lupus pleuritis; (9) infection; and (10) paragonimiasis. A simple mnemonic for this is **"reach tulip."**

Pleural fluid triglyceride levels need not be measured routinely but should be obtained if a chylous effusion is suspected. **Triglyceride levels** above 110 mg/dL suggest chylothorax. In this case, chyle, a milky emulsion formed in the lymphatics from fat droplets, has accumulated in the pleural space. The etiology is usually disruption of the thoracic duct by penetrating or blunt trauma, surgery, lymphoma, cancer, or granulomatous diseases. Up to 30% of **chylothoraces** may be idiopathic. Not all chylothoraces are milky, and often, fluid is serous, bloody, or turbid. Nutritional depletion is common if effusions are chronic. **Pseudochylous** effusions, on the other hand, are often milky, long-standing effusions usually associated with pleural thickening (such as those that occur after several years in patients with trapped lung or rheumatoid disease). Very high values of cholesterol (and sometimes triglycerides) are measured in the pleural fluid. Lipoprotein electrophoresis may be necessary to confirm the diagnosis if **cholesterol** crystals are not identified in the pleural fluid sediment microscopically.

Management of Pleural Effusions

If **thoracentesis** does not confirm the clinical diagnosis, particularly for exudates, additional evaluation is warranted. **Closed-needle pleural biopsy** is indicated if malignancy or tuberculosis is suspected. Otherwise, thoracoscopic biopsy is most likely to yield the diagnosis. **Thoracoscopy** may also be desirable to obtain satisfactory pleural tissue for culture, particularly in view of the increasing incidence of multidrug resistance tuberculosis. **Empiric therapy** of patients with unconfirmed pleural tuberculosis is rarely warranted and may result in misdiagnosis, drug resistance, or delay in detecting other diseases such as pleural carcinomatosis or malignant mesothelioma.

Patients with **recurrent effusions** should be considered for pleurodesis if symptoms resolve after initial large-volume thoracentesis or if rapidly recurrent, disabling malignant effusion is suspected. Talc is currently the most successful pleurodesis agent available. Thoracoscopic **pleurodesis** should probably be reserved for patients with higher Karnofsky performance levels and estimated survival beyond 3 months. Success of **talc** pleurodesis in patients with malignant effusions is usually greater than 90%.

Most patients with **complicated parapneumonic effusions** respond well to chest tube drainage, although patients with multiple loculations or fibrinous adhesions may warrant thoracoscopic drainage. **Chest tubes** should be placed in dependent areas, and complete lung reexpansion should be assured. If the clinical response is unsatisfactory (persistent fever or leukocytosis), the patient may be progressing towards empyema, and **surgical drainage** may be necessary.

Empyema is defined as pus or bacteria in the pleural space (grossly purulent fluid on thoracentesis, more than 50,000 WBC/mm^3, or presence of bacteria on Gram stain or culture). Empyemas often represent the final stage of a complicated parapneumonic effusion and are described as being in the exudative, fibropurulent, or organized stage. During the organized stage, a thick **"pleural peel"** may form over the parietal and visceral pleura, impeding lung expansion. Progression from early to later **stages of empyema** can be very rapid. Because morbidity and mortality are directly related to delays in treatment, empyemas should be treated immediately upon diagnosis; hence the ancient surgical edict, "the sun should never set on a suspected empyema." Although large-bore **chest tube drainage** (at least 32 Fr) and rapid institution of intravenous antibiotics are the initial procedures of choice, expert pleural disease or thoracic surgical consultation is usually warranted, and consideration should always be given to additional therapeutic alternatives such as **thoracoscopic drainage** with lysis of adhesions, **rib resection** with open drainage, or **decortication**. Occasionally, image-guided chest tube insertion is warranted to drain small loculations. In these cases, intrapleural instillation of **fibrinolytics** may be helpful to break up loculations and facilitate drainage. Further studies are needed to best determine the ideal indication for each of the above treatment modalities.

Hemothorax is usually the result of penetrating or blunt chest trauma. Occasionally, hemothorax results from laceration of the lung or intercostal vessels during thoracentesis or closed-needle pleural biopsy. Immediate large-bore (usually 36 Fr) **chest tube insertion** allows evacuation of blood, quantification of the amount of blood lost, determination of persistent bleeding that warrants surgical exploration, and potential avoidance of subsequent empyema or fibrothorax. Concomitant **antibiotic** administration is usually warranted, and any blood removed from the pleural space can be autotransfused (the Pleur-Evac and Sherwood chest drainage devices are available with autotransfusion units). Even after the bleeding has been controlled by tube thoracostomy, retained blood clots may cause prolonged fever. In these cases, eventual thoracoscopic or open **surgical exploration** should be considered.

Diagnosis of Pneumothorax

Spontaneous pneumothoraces are considered idiopathic in otherwise healthy individuals without other underlying lung disease. Pneumothorax size is inaccurately measured using radiographs, so therapeutic decisions should be based on clinical status. Computed tomographic (CT) scans are helpful when they reveal localized or extensive bullous lung disease, blebs, or adhesions between the lung and chest wall. In young persons with spontaneous pneumothoraces, apical **blebs** (small elevations of visceral pleura usually less than 1 cm in diameter) are common.

Secondary pneumothoraces result from trauma (blunt or penetrating), **iatrogenic** causes (as a result of mechanical ventilation, central line placement, nerve blocks, bronchoscopic lung biopsy or brushing, thoracentesis, closed-needle pleural biopsy, or percutaneous needle aspiration of a lung nodule), or rupture of blebs, bullae, or cysts in patients with underlying **lung diseases** (such as chronic obstructive pulmonary disease (COPD), cystic fibrosis, and *Pneumocystis carinii* pneumonia). Other causes of pneumothorax include tuberculosis and catamenial pneumothorax.

Management of Pneumothorax

Therapeutic alternatives for patients with pneumothorax include simple observation, aspiration, chest tube insertion with or without pleurodesis, and surgical intervention (thoracoscopy or open thoracotomy with resection of blebs and bullae, pleurectomy, or pleurodesis). Pneumothorax size is inaccurately measured using imaging studies, and size does not necessarily correlate with physical signs or symptoms, so that management decisions should be based on symptoms, risk of clinical deterioration, and overall clinical setting. It is noteworthy that in the United States no consensus exists regarding ideal management.

Most experts agree that the **risk of recurrence** increases with each pneumothorax event. Therefore, patients with recurrences, with life-threatening symptoms at first occurrence, or with prolonged air leaks despite chest tube drainage should probably be considered for aggressive treatment and pleurodesis. **Pleurodesis** can be achieved by instillation of sclerosing agents through the chest tube. If the patient is a satisfactory surgical candidate, however, consideration should be given to definitive treatment by open surgical or thoracoscopic resection of blebs and bullae and pleurodesis. Patients with **cystic fibrosis** who are potential lung transplant candidates should probably not undergo chemical or talc pleurodesis unless absolutely necessary.

Diagnosis of Pleural Thickening and Fibrothorax

Pleural thickening usually results from chronic pleural disease, including recurrent pleurisy, tuberculosis, empyema, hemothorax, collagen vascular and other inflammatory diseases, benign asbestos-related disease, benign fibrous mesothelioma, malignant mesothelioma, and pleural carcinomatosis. Clinical suspicion of malignancy, including malignant mesothelioma, may warrant thoracoscopic pleural biopsy. Thoracoscopy will also be helpful for staging the extent of disease in **malignant mesothelioma**. Closed-needle pleural biopsy should be done carefully in the absence of pleural fluid because of the risk of penetrating adjacent lung parenchyma. CT scanning is usually indicated to determine the extent of pleural abnormalities, and pulmonary function testing may be warranted to measure physiologic impairment.

Management of Pleural Thickening and Fibrothorax

Conservative measures usually suffice, but **decortication** may be warranted in the presence of benign pleural disease accompanied by symptoms and physiologic evidence of **restrictive ventilatory impairment** (decrease in forced vital capacity and overall lung volumes), particularly in cases of chronic empyema where a thick pleural peel inhibits lung expansion.

☆ Clinical Pearls

- In addition to chylothorax, other pleural effusions related to impaired lymphatics include lymphoma, pleural carcinomatosis, lymphangiomatosis (which often entails the association of chylothorax, interstitial lung disease, and pneumothorax usually in women of child-bearing age), and yellow nail syndrome (which usually entails straw-colored exudate and peripheral edema with or without discolored nails).
- Paramalignant effusions (nonmalignant effusions in a patient with cancer) may be caused by drug reactions, radiation pleuritis, postirradiation mediastinal fibrosis with lymphatic or vascular obstruction, organ failure, or any of the many diseases responsible for exudative or transudative pleural effusions.
- Pleural effusions from postcardiac injury syndrome (Dressler's syndrome) occur anywhere from 1 day to 3 months after heart surgery, pacemaker insertion, chest trauma, or myocardial infarction. Symptoms usually include pleuritic chest pain, low-grade temperature, and dyspnea. Although usually self-limiting, treatment may

require multiple thoracenteses, antiinflammatory medications, corticosteroids, or pleurodesis.

- Pulmonary embolism or infarction may cause exudative effusions that are not always bloody.
- To effectively manage patients with pleural effusions, develop a differential diagnosis before and after thoracentesis, and attempt to explain a reason for the effusion.

Heard on the Wards

Question: What is the significance of mesothelial cells in pleural fluid?

Answer: Mesothelial cells are single-layered cells with abundant surface microvillae that trap hyaluronic acid–rich glycoproteins. In addition to serving as lubricants between pleural surfaces, they probably have a role in fluid transport, fibrinolysis, and malignant transformation. Exfoliated cells are commonly found in pleural effusions, but patients with empyema or with complicated parapneumonic and tuberculous effusions have a paucity of mesothelial cells in their pleural fluid (less than 1%). Hyperreactive mesothelial cells can be confused with malignant cells.

Question: What is the significance of an elevated pleural fluid pH?

Answer: You mean higher than "normal" (7.65)? This is a frequent and relevant error. If the pH is elevated, the technique of fluid collection and measurement should be questioned. For example, if the fluid was collected and run aerobically, the CO_2 will diffuse into the atmosphere, and the pH will rise. Pleural fluid should therefore be collected and run anaerobically similar to an arterial blood gas.

Question: When should I not place a chest tube for a complicated parapneumonic effusion?

Answer: This is a tough question. Some believe that not all complicated parapneumonic effusions require drainage, especially if the patient has pneumococcal pneumonia. Also, what counts is drainage, not necessarily how its drained, so even thoracentesis with total evacuation of the pleural effusion may suffice in many instances. Effusions with a pH of less than 7.0 should probably be drained. If the pleural fluid pH is between 7.2 and 7.0, and drops further on subsequent thoracentesis done 6 to 12 hours later, particularly if symptoms have not improved and

TABLE 8-1. Differential Diagnosis of Pleural Effusion

Diagnosis	Color	Predominant cell type	pH	Diagnostic features	Comments
TRANSUDATES					
CHF, cirrhosis, nephrotic syndrome, peritoneal dialysis (PD), urinothorax	Straw-colored	Lymphocytes, mesothelial cells, mononuclear cells	>7.40	PD—glucose >300 mg/dL Urinothorax—pleural/serum creatine ratio >1 Ammonia odor	Cirrhosis—right-sided >70% Urinothorax—effusion ipsilateral to obstructed kidney
EXUDATES					
Infection					
Parapneumonic (uncomplicated)	Turbid/purulent	PMNs	Usually >7.30	LDH <500 U/L Glucose >60 mg/dL	Resolves with appropriate antibiotics
Empyema	White	PMNs	<7.10 or 0.3 U <art pH	Glucose <40 mg/dL, LDH >1,000, Pus, Positive Gram stain or culture	Requires antibiotics and immediate drainage
Tuberculosis	Straw-colored/serosanguinous	Acute-PMNs; chronic-lymphocytes	Always <7.40 20% <7.30	Positive AFB smear, culture, ADA >70 U/L in patients without empyema or rheumatoid arthritis	Pleural fluid/tissue diagnostic in >90%, often < 5% mesothelial cells
Amebic liver abscess	Anchovy-colored	PMNs		Positive amebic gel diffusion test	Requires tube drainage
Aspergillosis	Black	Lymphocytes, mesothelial cells		Positive pleural fluid culture	Brown clumps, hyphae suggestive
Malignancy					
Lung cancer Breast cancer	Serous/bloody	Lymphocytes, macrophages, mesothelial cells	> or <7.30	Positive cytology/pleural tissue	CEA, CD-15, B72.3, EMA are all positive in adenocarcinoma

Diagnosis	Color	Predominant cell type	pH	Diagnostic features	Comments
Lymphoma	Serous	Few lymphocytes	>7.30 20% <7.30	Positive cytology/ flow cytometry	Often responds to chemotherapy
Mesothelioma	Serous/bloody/ viscous	Mononuclear cells	<7.30	Tissue diagnosis	Increased hyaluronic acid supportive; CEA, CD15, B72.3, EMA are all negative
Connective Tissue Disease					
SLE	Serous/bloody	PMNs	Usually >7.30 20% <7.30	Positive LE cells	Low complement Pleural ANA >1:160 Increased immune complexes
Rheumatoid arthritis	Yellow-green	Lymphocytes	<7.20	Glucose <30 mg/dL	RF >1:320, low complement
General					
Pulmonary embolism	Straw-colored/ bloody	PMNs	>7.30	None	Bloody effusion is not a contra-indication to anticoagulation
Pancreatitis	Serosanguinous/ bloody	PMNs	7.30–7.35	Pleural fluid/serum amylase >1	60% are left-sided effusions
Chylothorax	Milky/bloody/ turbid/serous	Lymphocytes	>7.40	Pleural triglycerides >110 mg/dL Presence of chylomicrons	Trauma, surgery, or lymphoma
Esophageal rupture	Early/serous Late/turbid/purulent	PMNs	Early >7.30 Late <7.30	pH 6.00, elevated amylase	Gross food particles may be present
Asbestos exposure	Serosanguinous	PMNs, monos, eosinophils	>7.30	Presumptive	Often recurrent

ADA, Adenosine deaminase; AFB, acid-fast bacillus; ANA, antinuclear antibody; CEA, carcinoembryonic antigen; CHF, congestive heart failure; EMA, Epithelial membrane antigen; LDH, lactate dehydrogenase; PMN, polymorphonuclear leukocyte; RF, rheumatoid factor; SLE, systemic lupus erythematosis.

the patient is persistently febrile or has an elevated WBC, a chest tube is probably warranted.

Question: When should I consider pleurodesis for patients with malignant pleural effusions?
Answer: You should consider it in all patients with malignant effusions, but it is warranted only if you think the patient will live for 3 months or more. In addition, you should demonstrate that the patient has symptomatic improvement after thoracentesis, that the recurrence of symptoms is actually attributable to the recurrent effusion, and that the patient has disease that is unlikely to be rapidly responsive to systemic therapy.

Question: What is a catamenial pneumothorax?
Answer: These are spontaneous, recurrent pneumothoraces that occur in women around the time of their menstrual period. By the way, if you don't ask, you'll never diagnose one. Symptoms are often mild. Although the most frequently discovered pleural abnormalities are apical blebs, some women may have focal pleuropulmonary implants of endometriosis. Treatment includes bleb resection, pleurodesis, or suppression of ovulation. Oh yes, the word *catamenial* comes from the Greek words *kata* ("according to") and *menios* ("moon"), and has nothing to do with felines.

Question: What does having a "trapped lung" mean?
Answer: Don't be fooled into thinking that this is an iatrogenic pneumothorax or spontaneous bronchopleural fistula. Failure of the lung to fill the pleural cavity after large-volume thoracentesis may be due to the presence of a thick visceral peel; tethering of the lung at its base or apex; inadequate elevation of the space-occupying ipsilateral hemidiaphragm after lobectomy; or substantial pleuropulmonary adhesions resulting from pleural carcinomatosis or chronic benign pleurisy. Such trapped lungs will usually not expand, even after chest tube drainage, and should probably be managed conservatively. Decortication is sometimes warranted in symptomatic patients with benign disease.

Recommended Reading

Ashbaugh DG. Empyema thoracic: factors influencing morbidity and mortality. Chest 1991;99:1162–1165.
Delay in treatment resulted in greater morbidity. Decortication was more effective than open drainage in this particular study.

Baumann MH, Strange C. The clinician's perspective on pneumothorax management. Chest 1997;112:822–828.
A review of different practice patterns and physician preferences.

Bouros D, Schiza S, Patsourakis G, Chalkiadakis G, Panagou P, Siafakas NM. Intrapleural streptokinase versus urokinase in the treatment of complicated parapneumonic effusions. Am J Respir Crit Care Med 1997;155:291–295.
Higher cost and allergy potential of streptokinase make urokinase the agent of choice when intrapleural fibrinolytics are warranted.

Carter EJ, Ettensohn DB. Catamenial pneumothorax. Chest 1990;98:713–716.
A summary of epidemiology, clinical features, pathogenesis, and management alternatives.

Jannssen JP, Schramel FM, Sutedja TG, Cuesta MA, Postmus PE. Videothoracoscopic appearance of first and recurrent pneumothorax. Chest 1995;108:330–334.
Recurrence could not be predicted based on thoracoscopic findings alone.

Light RW, MacGregor MI, Luchsinger PC, et al. Pleural effusions: the diagnostic separation of transudates and exudates. Ann Intern Med 1972;77:507–513.
A landmark article.

Sahn SA. The pleura: state of the art. Am Rev Respir Dis 1988; 138:184–234.
Vintage Sahn. A must-read.

Valentine VG, Raffin TA. The management of chylothorax. Chest 1992;102:586–591.
A fine review of the anatomy of the thoracic lymphatic system and of pathogeneses, potential etiologies, and management alternatives.

II. PLEURAL PROCEDURES

9. THORACENTESIS

✣ Definition

Thoracentesis is percutaneous needle aspiration of pleural fluid from the pleural space.

❍ Indications

- To determine the etiology of pleural fluid accumulation.
- To relieve dyspnea, hypoxemia, and chest discomfort related to the accumulation of pleural fluid or blood.

● Contraindications

- Lack of patient cooperation or consent.
- Uncorrected coagulopathy.

❖ Equipment

Simple 2-inch **22-gauge and 18-gauge needles** are very useful when only 20 to 60 cm^3 of fluid must be obtained for diagnostic purposes. Avoiding large-bore needles and angiocatheters prevents potential morbidity from lung laceration, pneumothorax, and shearing off of the angiocatheter into the pleural cavity (Fig. 9-1).

The **Boutin needle** is a three-part stainless steel needle with a 3-mm outer canal and two-way stopcock (on/off), a sharp inner trocar, and a blunt inner trocar.

The **Argyle-Turkel safety needle** is a 9-cm-long, single-use, 8-Fr, graduated catheter mounted on a beveled, 16-gauge, hollow needle that houses a blunt-tipped, retractable canal and one-way safety valve.

◆ Techniques

Before

Informed consent should include the indication for thoracentesis, a simple review of potential management options dependent on the results of thoracentesis, and a description of potential complications and their treatment.

The chest radiographs are reviewed, and the chart is studied to detect bleeding abnormalities and allergy history, particularly to local anesthetics (lidocaine), povidone-iodine, or silk tape. Anxious patients benefit from administration of an anxiolytic such as midazolam. Atropine 0.5 to 1.2 mg by intramuscular injection can be given at least 30 minutes before the procedure to help prevent vasovagal reactions. Patients need not be NPO ("nothing by mouth").

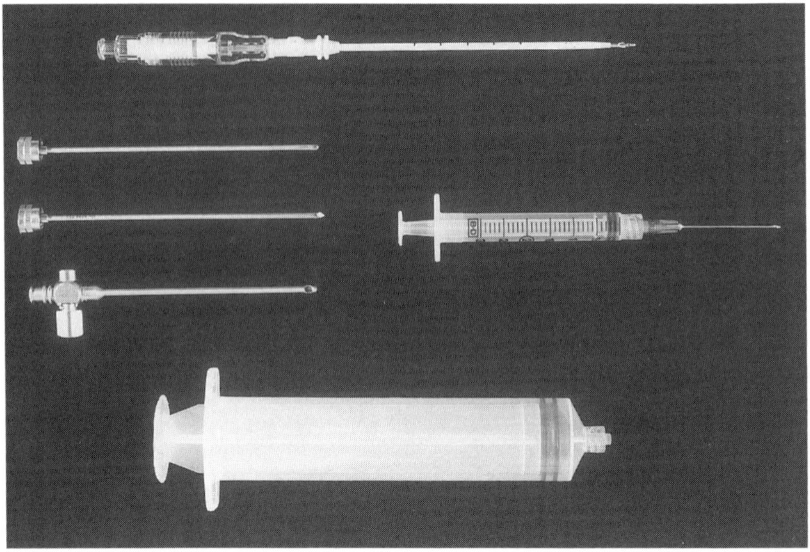

FIG. 9-1. Examples of instruments for thoracentesis. *From top to bottom:* Argyle-Turkel safety needle with attached angiocatheter, three-part Boutin pleural puncture needle with stopcock and both sharp and blunt inner trocars, 3-cm^3 syringe and 22-gauge needle, and simple 60-cm^3 syringe.

Thoracentesis is most easily performed with patients in the upright sitting position. This is easily achieved using an adjustable procedure chair, or by having the patient sit on the edge of the bed with legs dangling over the side and feet supported on a stool. An assistant should stand in front of the patient to monitor vital signs, provide reassurance, and keep patients from leaning too far forward. A bedside stand or table with a pillow on it may be used for the patient to rest his or her arms while sitting upright. The patient's chin is easily rested on crossed or folded hands. A towel should be placed around the patient's waist so that blood, povidone-iodine, or water does not drip onto slacks, skirts, or gowns (Fig. 9-2).

During

Careful examination of the posterior chest precedes selection of the target area. Both posterior hemithoraces are comparatively examined. Thoracentesis should be performed in an area of dullness to percussion, decreased breath sounds, and loss of tactile fremitus. Usually, a site two to four finger breadths below the tip of the scapula is selected.

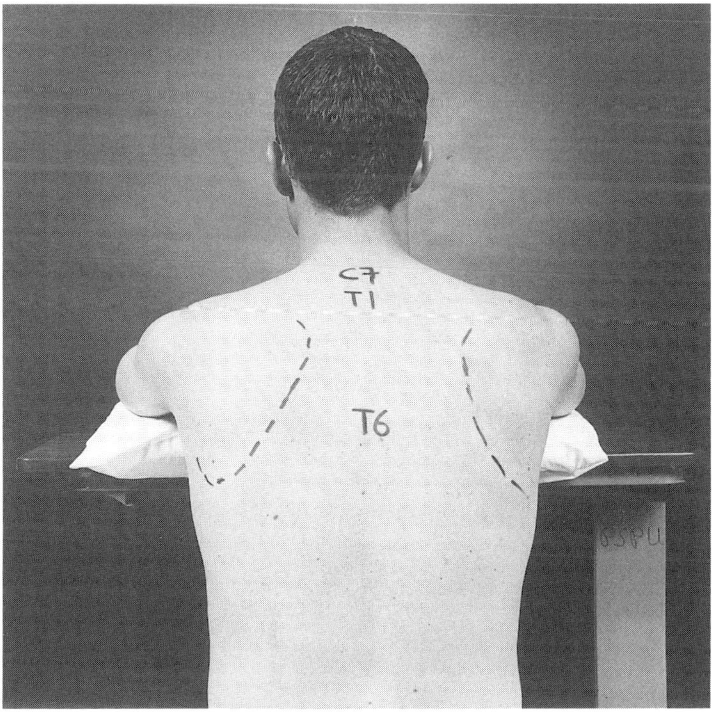

FIG. 9-2. Patient position for thoracentesis. Note how the shoulders are raised and the arms are pulled forward, resting comfortably on the table. This pulls the scapula laterally and upward to about the 6th intercostal space.

Skin disinfection is confined to the target area of thoracentesis. A wide preparation is unnecessary. Povidone-iodine solution is applied to the skin with sterile gauze, then blotted dry. Local anesthesia is provided using 1% or 2% lidocaine introduced through a short 25-gauge needle. First a large wheal is raised at the skin and subcutaneous tissues overlying the upper margin or the rib overlying the planned thoracentesis site (Fig. 9-3). Then, using a 2-in., 22-gauge needle and 3-cm^3 syringe, additional lidocaine is injected through the wheal perpendicularly and downward into the subcutaneous and intercostal tissues, with care taken to remain above the superior margin of the underlying rib. It is not necessary to intermittently aspirate during injection.

Once these tissues are infiltrated, another 3-cm^3 syringe containing lidocaine is used to access the pleural space. The needle is directed perpendicularly through the previously made needle track while maintaining gentle suction. When pleural fluid is

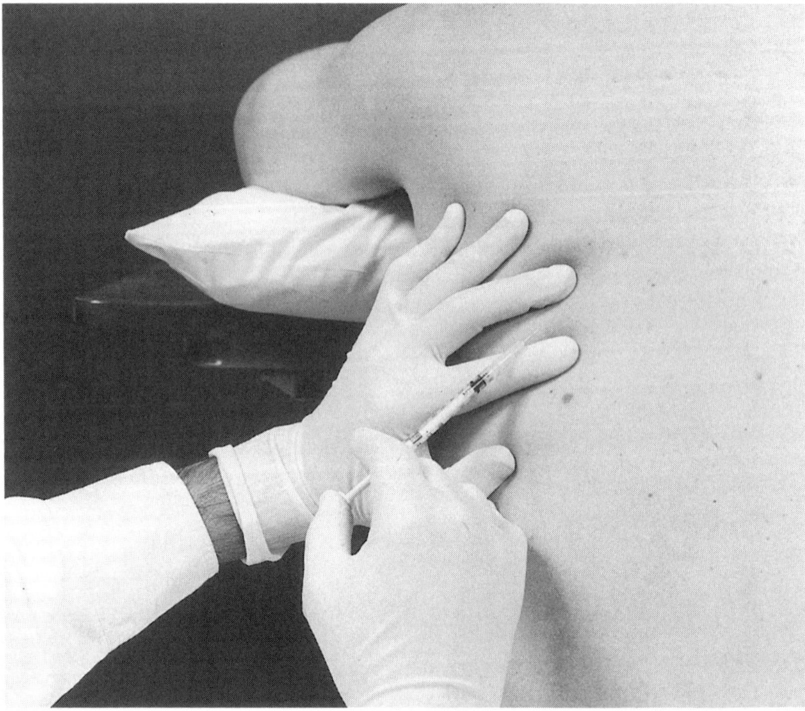

FIG. 9-3. The index and middle finger of the left hand are each placed on a rib above and below the area within the intercostal space chosen for thoracentesis.

aspirated, the needle is withdrawn slightly, and the parietal pleura is anesthetized. The needle can be redirected slightly inferiorly or superiorly to infiltrate a greater area. It is rarely necessary to inject lidocaine into rib periosteum (this is unnecessarily painful) or to "step" over the rib into the target intercostal space. All of the lidocaine in each syringe should be injected (Fig. 9-4).

A 22- or 18-gauge needle: For simple aspiration of a small amount of fluid (less than 120 cm^3), a 22-gauge needle attached to a 60-cm^3 syringe can be used. The pleural space is accessed, the syringe filled, and fluid sent for appropriate analyses. One cubic centimeter of fluid can be easily withdrawn from the syringe into an arterial blood gas syringe for pH analysis. Otherwise, an 18-gauge needle can be used, attached to a 20- to 60-cm^3 syringe via a three-way stopcock. After fluid is aspirated, it is injected back through the stopcock into an attached drainage bag. In this manner, the syringe is never removed from

a) b) c) d)

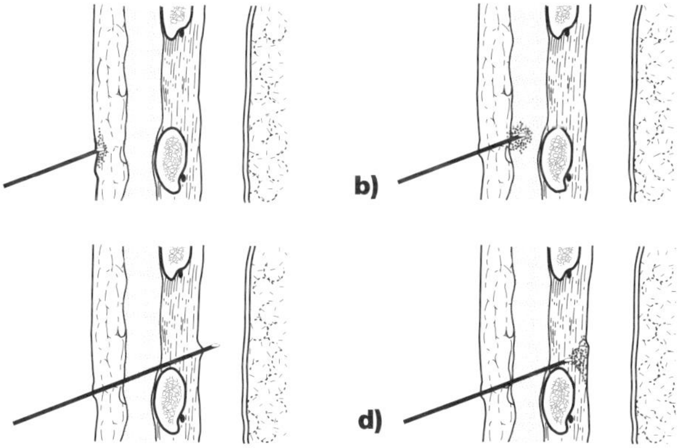

FIG. 9-4. Technique of thoracentesis. **(A)** A large subcutaneous wheal is raised using a small needle and lidocaine. **(B)** Injecting through the wheal while advancing the needle allows additional administration of local anesthetic into the intercostal tissues. **(C)** The pleura is penetrated, as confirmed by aspiration of a small amount of pleural fluid. **(D)** The needle is then pulled back slightly so that additional anesthetic can be injected onto the parietal pleural and surrounding tissues. Reinjecting through the large subcutaneous wheal and injecting the parietal pleural only once helps avoid pain.

the ensemble. Gentle aspiration is safer and better tolerated than rapid suction using high negative pressures. Care must be taken, however, to avoid moving the needle too far into the pleural space since the sharp needle can easily puncture lung or rip intrapleural adhesions.

The Boutin needle (Richard Wolf Inc.): After making a small stab incision through the skin and superficial intercostal tissues using a no. 11 scalpel, the cannula and sharp inner trocar are inserted. Before penetrating through the parietal pleura, however, the sharp trocar is replaced by the blunt trocar. The needle is inserted using constant but gentle forward pushing and rotation motion. Penetration through the parietal pleura can be felt by a loss of resistance and small "give" as the needle advances. Sometimes a light pop can be heard. The patient is asked to hum, at which time the blunt trocar is removed, the stopcock turned to the off position, and a 60-cm^3 syringe attached to the outer canal. The stopcock is then turned to the on position and fluid is gently aspirated. Following withdrawal of fluid for diagnostic studies, a vacutainer bottle is attached to the needle via a male-to-male metal adapter and 30-cm intravenous extension tubing with

Luer locks. The rate of fluid removal into the vacutainer is regulated by the stopcock.

The Argyle-Turkel safety needle (Sherwood Medical): This needle is inserted through the skin into the pleural cavity. During insertion through the intercostal tissues and parietal pleura, the inner cannula withdraws into the hollow shaft. Once through the pleura and into fluid, however, it automatically extends past the bevel, protecting the lung from further needle penetration. As the inner cannula retracts, a color indicator turns red. As it extends again, the indicator turns green. Once in place, the needle is withdrawn leaving the polyurethane catheter in the pleural space. Fluid is withdrawn using the attached three-way stopcock.

After

The skin is cleaned of blood or povidone-iodine and a small, sterile dressing applied. Sometimes fluid or blood may ooze from the wound; it would be unfortunate for this to stain the patient's shirt or gown. Later, the dressing can be removed or replaced with a Band-aid. Two-view **chest radiographs** (posteroanterior and lateral) are warranted to ascertain the effect of the amount of fluid removed on mediastinal shift or diaphragm inversion, visualize possible atelectasis or pulmonary infiltrates on the side of the effusion, detect an increase of pleural effusion that would be suggestive of iatrogenic hemothorax, and detect a procedure-related pneumothorax.

Pleural fluid should be sent for **selective laboratory studies** based on the differential diagnosis established prior to thoracentesis and clinical suspicion. Routine studies usually include (1) cytology; (2) microbiology including bacterial, mycobacterial, and fungal smears and cultures; (3) chemistry including lactate dehydrogenase (LDH) and protein, and glucose; (4) hemoglobin, white blood count, and differential; and (5) pH (performed immediately on fluid aspirated into a blood gas syringe and run through the arterial blood gas analyzer, not sent to the chemistry laboratory). Additional **specific studies** may include (1) triglycerides or lipid profile (triglycerides, cholesterol, and chylomicrons) although most laboratories will not run these routinely; (2) hematocrit; (3) amylase; and (4) cholesterol or bilirubin.

The ideal thoracentesis procedure note should include (1) the indication for thoracentesis (e.g., dyspneic patients with pleural effusion of unknown etiology); (2) the site of thoracentesis (along, lateral to, or medial to the midscapular line) and which intercostal space and hemithorax were accessed; (3) the amount of fluid removed; (4) a description of the technique and needle used; (5) a gross description of the fluid (dark yellow or straw-colored serous, serosanguinous, grossly bloody); (6) the pH value of the fluid; (7) the patient's tolerance of the procedure and whether any adverse events occurred; and (8) results of the postprocedure chest radiograph.

▼ Complications

- Hemothorax may occur from inadvertent laceration of an intercostal vessel or lung. Avoidance of the neurovascular bundle along the inferior margin of the rib and gradual insertion of the needle into the pleural space while gently maintaining traction on the syringe will prevent this complication.
- Vasovagal reactions associated with bradycardia, systemic hypotension, nausea, and diaphoresis can occur in young, anxious patients, and in patients who have not eaten before thoracentesis. Usually, a vasovagal reaction prompts immediate cessation of the procedure to place patients in the reverse Trendelenburg position. There is no evidence that premedication with atropine prevents this complication. Careful monitoring of pulse and blood pressure during thoracentesis helps to detect vasovagal reactions as they occur.
- Pneumothorax may occur if the needle penetrates the visceral pleura or if ambient air is inadvertently introduced into the pleural cavity. This can be avoided by having the patient hum loudly at any time when the inserted needle is open to atmospheric pressure.
- Reexpansion pulmonary edema is believed to be caused by increased endothelial permeability resulting from alveolar-capillary disruption and ischemia-reperfusion injury. Although its true frequency is unknown, consequences include prolonged hypoxemia, unilateral or bilateral pulmonary infiltrates on chest radiograph, and respiratory insufficiency.
- Persistent cough often occurs as increasing amounts of fluid are removed, irritating the reexpanding lung. If patients cough forcefully or persistently, the needle should be removed and thoracentesis stopped because of the risk of lung perforation.
- Soft tissue infection along the needle tract or bacterial contamination of the pleural space is rare if sterile technique is used for thoracentesis.

☆ Clinical Pearls

- Proper patient positioning is essential to enhance pleural fluid flow posteriorly and inferiorly, and widen the intercostal space.
- As fluid is removed, the lung expands, pushing fluid toward the needle. Needle insertion into the lowest point of the effusion, therefore, is usually unnecessary.
- Thoracentesis can be painless if you create a large cutaneous wheal, generously use local anesthesia in the subcutaneous tissues and parietal pleura, and avoid "stepping" over the rib.
- Usually, 60 to 100 cm^3 of fluid is enough for most laboratory analyses and a satisfactory diagnostic yield from cytologic examination. If removing additional fluid into a vacuum container bottle or a collection bag, this extra fluid can also be sent to the cytology laboratory for analysis.
- The negative pressure applied by most commercially available vacuum container bottles is at least –300 cm of water.

Heard on the Wards

Question: How can I minimize cough and patient discomfort during thoracentesis?

Answer: Cough or chest discomfort are usually related to rapid reexpansion of collapsed underlying lung. These are minimized by (1) explaining to the patient what is happening; (2) avoiding the use of a vacuum container bottle, which exerts high negative pressures and causes rapid evacuation of pleural fluid; (3) limiting large-volume thoracentesis to less than 1,500 cm^3 unless pleural pressures are being measured using a pleural manometer.

Question: How do I avoid reexpansion pulmonary edema?

Answer: It is likely this complication can be avoided by removing fluid slowly, limiting the amount of fluid withdrawn to less than 1,500 cm^3 at one time, or measuring pleural pressures during thoracentesis and ceasing the procedure if pleural pressure falls to 20 cm H_2O or less.

Question: What local anesthetics should be used and how much is enough?

Answer: Pleural procedures can and should be painless. Lidocaine hydrochloride (Xylocaine) usually assures effective and immediate local anesthesia at a dose of 300 mg (15 mL of 2% solution). Doses greater than 7 mg/kg can result in blurred vision, tremors, dizziness, convulsions, or cardiovascular toxicity. Hypersensitivity reactions are rare. Bupivacaine (Marcaine) lasts longer and is about four times more potent and more toxic than lidocaine. Particularly useful for local infiltration of incision sites during thoracoscopy, the maximal single dose of bupivacaine should not exceed 200 mg (80 mL of 0.25% solution).

Question: What is a "dry tap?"

Answer: A dry tap represents failure to obtain fluid during attempted thoracentesis. Dry taps are not true complications of thoracentesis because they can occur when pleural fluid is not present, as well as when the needle is misdirected into an area without fluid. If the dry tap occurs because the needle is directed

✔ Procedural Guidelines: Thoracentesis

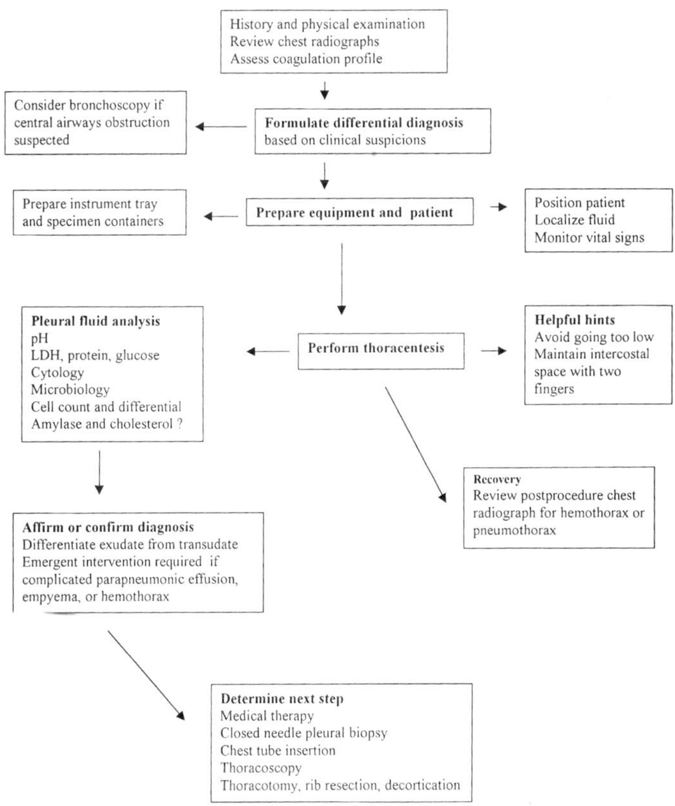

outside of the pleural space, such as into the diaphragm, liver, or spleen, it would be classified as a true complication (one that I, personally, prefer to avoid). Occasionally fluid cannot be withdrawn because the needle is obstructed by blood clot, pus, thick coagulum, or fibrinous debris. Other dry taps can result in pneumothorax or hemothorax from inadvertent laceration of the lung or intercostal vessels.

Question: How do I avoid a dry tap?

Answer: Dry taps are avoided by using careful technique, examining the patient diligently, carefully localizing the pleural effusion, searching to differentiate fluid from pleural thickening or consolidated lung based on interpretation of imaging studies, and judiciously using pleural ultrasonography. It is noteworthy that blood, pus, and fibrinous debris often cause difficulties in the interpretation of ultrasound images, so that an "exploratory" thoracentesis may be warranted even when the sonographic appearance is uncertain.

Recommended Reading

American College of Physicians. Diagnostic thoracentesis and pleural biopsy in pleural effusions. Ann Intern Med 1985;103:799–802.

A position paper by the health and policy committee of the ACP. Also states that patients with unexplained exudates have a 20% probability of presenting with malignancy at a later date.

Atwater EC. Morrill Wyman and the aspiration of acute pleural effusions, 1850. Bull Hist Med 1972;46:235–256.

Great reading for history buffs.

Jenkins DW, McKinney MK, Szpak MW, Booker JL. Veress needle in the pleural space. South Med J 1983;76:1383–1385.

Originally designed to induce pneumoperitoneum for peritoneoscopy, its use for thoracentesis was originally described in this article.

Lewis C, Colt HG. Pleural effusions. From thoracentesis to thoracoscopy. Physician Assist J 1996;20:68–83.

This article enables one to walk through the process.

Light RW, Jenkinson SG, Minh VD, George RB. Observations on pleural fluid pressures as fluid is withdrawn during thoracentesis. Am Rev Respir Dis 1980;121:799–804.

Increasingly negative pleural pressures during thoracentesis may signify reexpansion pulmonary edema. Pressures become more negative as additional (greater than 100 cm) fluid is removed.

Timby J, Zeilender S, Glauser FL. Mechanical causes of pulmonary edema. Chest 1990;98:973–979.

A summary of the pathogenesis and clinical presentations of postobstructive, reexpansion, and over-distention pulmonary edema.

10. CLOSED-NEEDLE PLEURAL BIOPSY

❖ Definition

Closed-needle pleural biopsy is percutaneous sampling of the parietal pleura using a needle that is inserted through the posterior chest wall.

❍ Indications

- Usually performed after an initial thoracentesis has been nondiagnostic.
- To improve diagnostic yield at the time of initial thoracentesis in patients presenting with unexplained pleural effusions or pleural thickening, particularly when pleural carcinomatosis or tuberculosis is highly suspected. After parietal pleura tissue for pathology and microbiology has been obtained, a thorough drainage of the pleural effusion is warranted unless thoracoscopy is being considered.

● Contraindications

- Lack of patient cooperation or consent.
- Uncorrected coagulopathy (particularly uremia, use of anticoagulant medication, or bleeding diathesis).
- Uncontrolled cough.
- Substantial localized skin disease such as pyoderma, herpes zoster, diffuse cutaneous infiltration with neoplasm.
- Insufficient pleural fluid to adequately and safely sample parietal pleura.
- Suspected empyema or complicated parapneumonic effusions because of risk of infecting the subcutaneous biopsy tract (although there is no recent scientific evidence to support this last contraindication).

❖ Equipment

The Cope Needle

This four-part needle includes an 11-gauge 3-mm diameter outer cannula, a 13-gauge hooked biopsy trocar, a hollow beveled trocar, and an inner stylet (Fig. 10-1). After placing a 10-cm^3 syringe on the hooked biopsy trocar, the inner stylet is inserted through the beveled trocar and both of these are inserted through the hollow cannula. This entire ensemble is then inserted along the superior margin of the rib into the pleural space. As the patient hums or holds his or her breath, the beveled trocar and inner stylet are removed simultaneously and a thumb is placed over

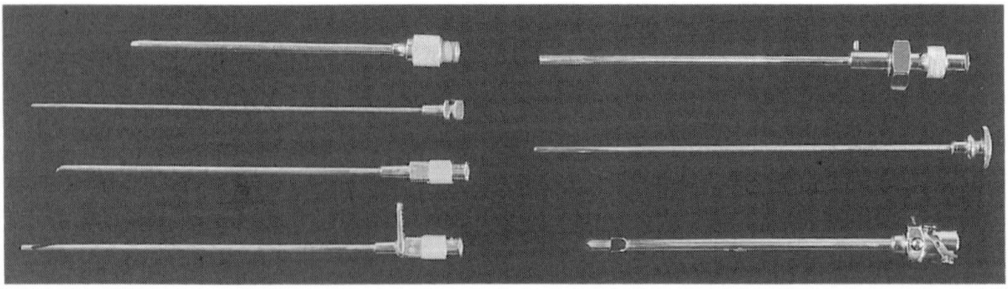

FIG. 10-1. Cope (left) and Abrams (right) pleural biopsy needles.

the outer cannula to prevent air entry. As the patient hums again, the hooked biopsy trocar and attached syringe are inserted through the cannula into the pleural space. Some pleural fluid is aspirated to confirm position. The perpendicular tab on the biopsy trocar indicates the direction of the distal biopsy hook or curette. The ensemble is withdrawn gently while the distal tip of the needle is tilted 10 to 45 degrees downward with pressure maintained on the needle and pleural tissues. The resistance felt indicates that the curette has "caught" the parietal pleural and intercostal muscle. While maintaining gentle traction on the biopsy trocar, the outer canal is rotated and advanced with the other hand to shear off the pleural specimen in the curette. The biopsy trocar is then withdrawn, with care taken to rapidly place a finger over the outer canal and to not catch one's thumb on the curette. Specimens should be taken with the perpendicular tab facing downward to avoid catching the neurovascular bundle (Fig. 10-2).

The Abrams Needle

This three-part needle consists of a 4-mm-diameter outer cannula with a beveled notch proximal to its tip, a hollow inner cannula, and an inner stylet (see Fig. 10-1). The cutting action of the inner canal as it is rotated samples the pleura. The stylet is placed in the inner cannula, which is inserted into the outer cannula and locked in place by twisting it clockwise. The entire ensemble is inserted into the pleural space. The stylet is removed, and a 20-cm^3 syringe is attached in its place to the outer cannula. The hexagonal grip of the inner cannula is twisted counterclockwise so that the beveled notch is oriented downward (the indicator knob points in the direction of the notch). The ensemble is then gently withdrawn while maintaining pressure and tilting the distal tip of the needle 10 to 45 degrees downward. When resistance is felt, parietal pleura has been caught in the notch.

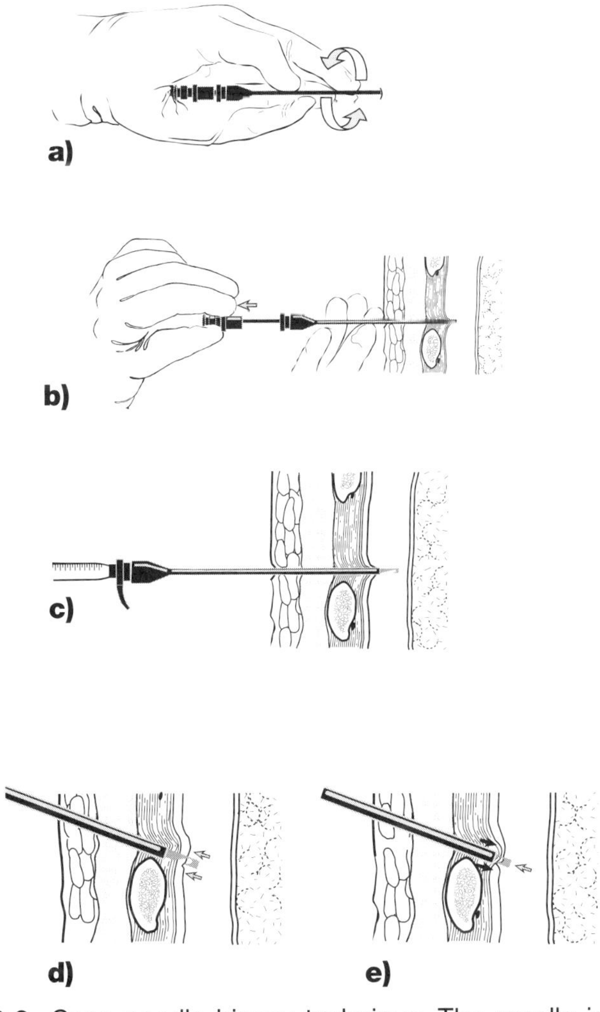

FIG. 10-2. Cope needle biopsy technique. The needle is inserted through a small stab incision using a rotating forward pushing motion **(A)**. Once in the pleural space, the inner trocar is removed while the patient hums or exhales **(B)**. Pleural fluid can be aspirated by attaching a syringe to the outer cannula, confirming entry into the pleural space. A syringe is attached to the biopsy curette that has been inserted through the outer cannula **(C)**. A small amount of fluid is again aspirated, and the entire ensemble is withdrawn as traction is maintained on the biopsy curette as it hooks onto parietal pleura **(D)**. While maintaining traction on the biopsy curette, the outer cannula is rotated and gently pushed back into the pleural space, shearing off the biopsy specimen caught on the curette **(E)**.

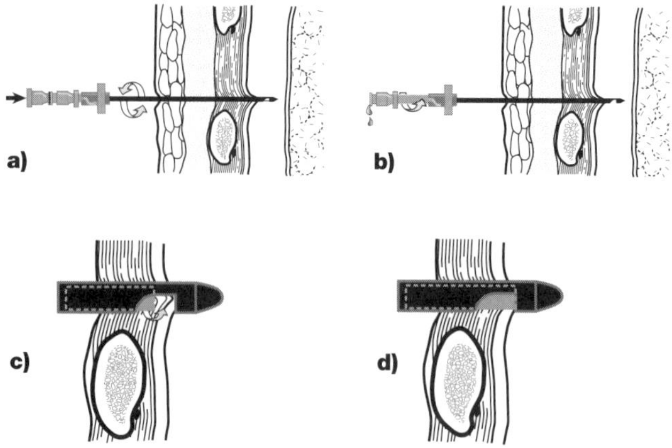

FIG. 10-3. Abrams needle biopsy technique. The needle is inserted through a small stab incision into the pleural space using a gentle rotating forward movement **(A)**. If the patient hums as the stylet is removed, pleural fluid will be evacuated **(B)**. To avoid pneumothorax from air entry during inspiration, place a syringe onto the inner cannula. The hexagonal grip of the inner cannula is twisted counterclockwise so that the beveled notch is oriented downward. The ensemble is then gently withdrawn until resistance is felt and the parietal pleura is caught in the notch **(C)**. By rotating the hexagonal grip clockwise, the beveled opening is closed, shearing the specimen off into the cannula **(D)**. The entire needle is then withdrawn from the pleural space.

The hexagonal grip is rotated clockwise to close the beveled opening, and the entire ensemble is removed from the chest to remove the specimen. To avoid withdrawing the needle entirely, however, the notch can be reopened by turning the inner cannula once more counterclockwise after reinserting the ensemble 1 cm or so back into the pleural space, and aspirating the pleural specimen as well as a few milliliters of fluid into the syringe (Fig. 10-3).

Closed-Needle Pleural Biopsy Techniques

Before

Informed consent should include the indication for biopsy, a simple review of potential management options dependent on the results of the biopsy, and a description of potential complications and their treatment.

The patient's chest radiographs are examined, and the chart is reviewed to note results of previous thoracenteses, detect bleeding abnormalities, and elicit potential allergies to local anesthetics (lidocaine), povidone-iodine, or silk tape. Anxious patients often benefit from administration of an anxiolytic such as midazolam. Atropine 0.5 to 1.2 mg by intramuscular injection can be given at least 30 minutes before the procedure to help prevent vasovagal reactions. Patients need not be NPO ("nothing by mouth").

During

Biopsy is most easily performed with patients in the upright sitting position. This is easily achieved using an adjustable procedure chair, or by having patient sit on the edge of the bed with legs hanging over the side and feet supported on a stool. An assistant should stand in front of the patient to monitor vital signs as needed, to comfort the patient with soothing words of reassurance, and to keep the patient from leaning too far forward. A bedside stand or table with a pillow on it may be used for the patient to rest his or her arms while sitting upright. The patient's chin is rested on crossed or folded hands. A towel should be placed around the back of the patient's waist so that blood, povidone-iodine, or water does not drip down his or her clothing.

Careful examination of the posterior chest precedes selection of the target area. When the shoulders are raised and the arms are folded in front of the patient, the scapulae are pulled outward and above the 6th intercostal space. In the sitting, upright position, the diaphragm is approximately at the 8th posterior intercostal space, but can be higher in patients with volume loss, ascites, or obesity. Both posterior hemithoraces are comparatively examined. Biopsy should be performed in an area of dullness to percussion, decreased breath sounds, and loss of tactile fremitus. Usually, a site two to four finger breadths below the tip of the scapula is selected.

Skin disinfection is confined to the target area of needle biopsy. A wide preparation is unnecessary. Povidone-iodine solution should be applied to the skin using sterile gauze, then blotted dry. Local anesthesia is provided using 1% or 2% lidocaine introduced through a 25-gauge needle. First a large wheal is raised at the skin and subcutaneous tissues overlying the upper margin of the rib overlying the planned thoracentesis site. Then, using a 2-in., 22-gauge needle and 3-cm^3 syringe, additional lidocaine is injected through the wheal perpendicularly into the subcutaneous and intercostal tissues, with care taken to remain above the superior margin of the underlying rib. More generous anesthesia than for simple thoracentesis is warranted.

Once these tissues are infiltrated, another 3-cm^3 syringe containing lidocaine is used to access the pleural space. The needle is directed perpendicularly through the previously made needle track while maintaining gentle suction. When pleural fluid is aspirated, the needle is withdrawn slightly and the parietal pleura is anesthetized. The needle should be withdrawn slightly and redirected laterally, medially, inferiorly, and superiorly to infiltrate a greater area of parietal pleura and intercostal muscle. Sometimes it is helpful to inject lidocaine into the periosteum of the underlying rib. Estimate the distance between the skin and pleural cavity.

A small stab incision is made through the skin and superficial intercostal tissues using a no. 11 scalpel. The Cope needle is more fragile than the Abrams needle, so the Cope needle biopsy hook should be carefully examined for sharpness and to ensure that it does not bend over the hollow cannula. Both the Cope and the Abrams needles have been known to break. Biopsies can be obtained inferiorly, laterally, and medially (at the 6, 4, and 8 o'clock positions), but should not be obtained superiorly (at the 12 o'clock position) because of the risk of severing the intercostal bundles. A short 22-gauge needle can be used to remove specimens from the biopsy needle. Pleural specimens are placed in formalin for pathology and in saline solution for microbiology. Parietal pleura is usually white and attached to a small piece of red intercostal muscle. After all specimens have been obtained (ideally at least two samples for pathology and two samples for microbiology), pleural fluid can be removed using 60-cm^3 syringes and a stopcock or by connecting the needle to a vacutainer bottle. Patients who might require chest tubes or thoracoscopy should not be drained dry.

After

The skin should be cleaned of blood or povidone-iodine and a compressive sterile dressing applied for at least 24 hours. Two-view chest radiographs (posteroanterior and lateral) are warranted to detect an increase of pleural effusion that would be suggestive of iatrogenic hemothorax or to detect a procedure-related pneumothorax.

The ideal closed-needle biopsy procedure note should include (1) the indication for biopsy (e.g., patient with unilateral right-sided exudative, lymphocytic pleural effusion and positive purified protein derivative, or PPD); (2) the results of previous thoracentesis; (3) a description of the procedure, including the needle used, the site of biopsy (along, lateral to, or medial to the midscapular line), and which intercostal space and hemithorax were accessed; (4) the number of parietal pleural specimens obtained for pathology and microbiology; (5) the amount of pleural fluid removed; (6) the patient's tolerance of the procedure; (7) whether any adverse events occurred; and (8) the results of a postprocedure chest radiograph.

▼ Complications

- Pneumothorax related to introduction of a small amount of air during the procedure should be expected in up to 15% of instances. This is best avoided by making trocar and cannula changes rapidly, and by having patients hum or hold their breaths during these changes. Usually treatment is not necessary.
- Pneumothorax related to laceration of lung parenchyma and visceral pleural tears will usually cause symptoms such as cough, pleuritic chest discomfort, or dyspnea. A greater than 10% sized pneumothorax is usually present on chest radiographs. Tube thoracostomy is usually warranted to relieve symptoms and reexpand the lung. The complication is usually caused by faulty technique.
- Subcutaneous emphysema from a small pneumothorax or pneumomediastinum usually does not require treatment.
- Hemothorax can occur from inadvertent laceration of intercostal vessels or lung parenchyma. Careful technique helps to avoid this complication. Biopsies should never be obtained from areas of parietal pleura where intercostal vessels lie (directly below the inferior margin of the ribs, and directly within the middle of the intercostal space within 6 cm lateral to the spine posteriorly).
- Vasovagal reactions can probably be reduced by keeping this procedure pain-free.

☆ Clinical Pearls

- To assure satisfactory diagnostic yield, at least two specimens should be obtained for pathology and two specimens obtained for microbiology.
- The entrance site can be well maintained by applying pressure on the target intercostal space with two fingers of the non needle-holding hand. An assistant should remove specimens from the needle and place them in the appropriate containers for laboratory analysis.
- Closed-needle pleural biopsy can be a painless procedure if adequate anesthesia is applied to intercostal tissues, the parietal pleura, and the periosteum of each adjacent rib.

Heard on the Wards

Question: In case of cancer, does seeding of the biopsy tract occur?

Answer: Malignant seeding of the biopsy track has been described in patients with malignant mesothelioma, but it can often be avoided by the use of preventive external beam radiation therapy following biopsy.

Question: How do I avoid cutting myself with the curette of a Cope needle?

Answer: First of all, double-glove. Before you obtain your pleural specimen, ask the patient to take a deep breath and hold it; take the specimen, and ask the patient to hum in order to avoid aspirating air into the pleural space. Quickly withdraw the hooked biopsy trocar from within the outer cannula while rotating the perpendicular tab so that it faces upward while displacing your thumb downward and away from the open end of the outer cannula. Once the inner trocar is withdrawn, replace your thumb quickly over the open end of the outer cannula. Believe it or not, all this takes less than 10 seconds; we've timed it!

Question: Should patients not eat or drink for several hours before or after this procedure?

Answer: No. Food is fine, and may actually help avoid fainting spells.

Question: Can I perform a biopsy in the absence of pleural fluid?

Answer: Yes. Biopsies should be done very carefully, however, and probably only in areas of pleural thickening when pleural tuberculosis or malignancy is suspected. The yield is usually less than 50%, so a thoracoscopic biopsy may be the procedure of choice in these instances.

Question: What are the best indications for doing a closed-needle pleural biopsy?

Answer: The highest yields for needle biopsy are in patients with suspected granulomatous pleural disease; primarily tuberculosis (yields often between 50% and 70%) and pleural carcinomatosis (yields often between 40% and 50%). In these two diseases, parietal pleural involvement is usually widespread rather

✔ Procedural Guidelines: Closed-Needle Pleural Biopsy

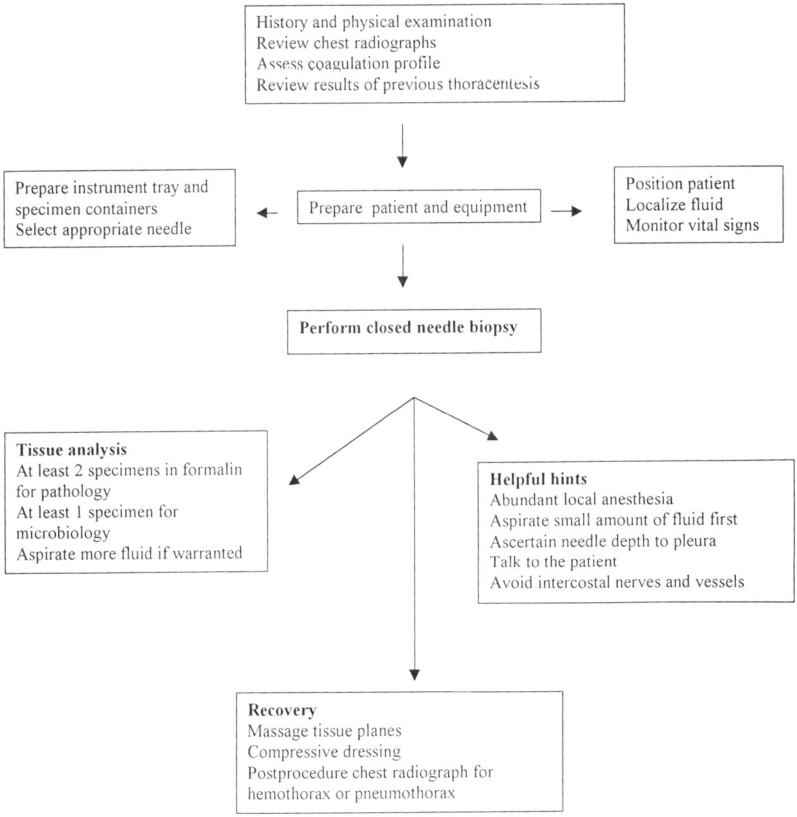

than focal. Granulomas on pleural tissue are usually indicative of tuberculosis, although fungal diseases, sarcoidosis, and, rarely, rheumatoid pleuritis should also be considered.

Recommended Reading

ATS position paper: Guidelines for thoracentesis and needle biopsy of the pleura. Am Rev Respir Dis 1989;140:257–258.
A to-the-point, one-page document.

Chang DB, Yang PC, Lee LN, Luh KT. Metallic weakness and breakage of Abrams pleural biopsy needle. Chest 1991;99:524.
Detachment of the trocar tip of the Abrams needle.

Cope C. New pleural biopsy needle. JAMA 1958;167:1107–1108.
The original description.

Eng P, Colt HG. Fracture of Cope's needle in closed pleural biopsy. Chest 1994;106:977–988.

If resistance is felt while withdrawing the curette, beware fracture of the needle!

Kirsch CM, Kroe M, Jensen WA, Kagawa FT, Wehner JH, Campagna AC. A modified Abrams needle biopsy technique. Chest 1995;108:982–986.

A clear description of use of the Abrams needle without multiple removals and reinsertions. Diagnostic sensitivity for pleural tuberculosis was 82%.

11. FINE-NEEDLE ASPIRATION BIOPSY

✤ Definition

Needle aspiration or biopsy of a parenchymal lung lesion using an 18- to 22-gauge needle inserted through the chest wall under fluoroscopic or computed tomography (CT) guidance. This procedure is also referred to as percutaneous needle aspiration (PCNA), transthoracic needle aspiration (TTNA), and transthoracic needle biopsy (TTNB).

❍ Indications

- To obtain histologic or cytologic material from an intrapulmonary lesion when other procedures such as bronchoscopy have failed, or when thoracotomy or thoracoscopy for diagnosis are not desirable.
- To obtain diagnostic material from an intrapulmonary lesion when the location or size of the lesion make percutaneous access more desirable than other invasive procedures such as bronchoscopy, thoracoscopy, or thoracotomy.
- Indications include multiple as well as solitary pulmonary nodules when either infection or neoplasm is suspected, especially if nodules are peripheral and less than 2 cm in diameter.
- The choice between fluoroscopic and CT guidance is usually a function of personal preference, experience, nodule location, and availability of equipment.

● Contraindications

- Lack of patient cooperation or consent.
- Uncorrected coagulopathy (particularly uremia, use of anticoagulant medication, or bleeding diathesis).
- Severe pulmonary hypertension (increased risk of bleeding).
- Advanced chronic obstructive lung disease with forced expiratory volume less than 1.0 L, particularly bullous emphysema. Consequences of possible pneumothorax must be weighed against the benefits of diagnosis.
- Patients with only one lung (post pneumonectomy). Consequences of possible pneumothorax must be weighed against the benefits of diagnosis.
- Lesions close to the mediastinum or hila (increased risk for bleeding).
- Abnormalities not easily seen using fluoroscopy can be approached using CT.

❖ **Equipment** (Figs. 11-1 and 11-2)

Turner Biopsy Needle (Cook Inc.)
This is a 15-cm-long, single-pass, 20-gauge needle with a beveled edge and a pointed inner stylet that protrudes approximately 0.4 cm beyond the tip of the needle. There are no marks on the needle itself, although a protective plastic outer sheath is marked at 1-cm intervals. Once the needle is inside the lesion, the inner stylet is removed and a syringe is attached to the proximal hub. Suction is applied as the needle is moved in and out of the lesion. The needle is withdrawn from the chest while maintaining suction. The specimen is flushed out of the needle onto specimen slides using air in the syringe.

Crown Biopsy Needle (Medi-tech)
This is a 20-cm-long, single-pass, 18-gauge needle (also known as a Franseen needle) with a three-pronged, crown-type tip and an inner stylet with a three-sided diamond-shaped tip. There are no

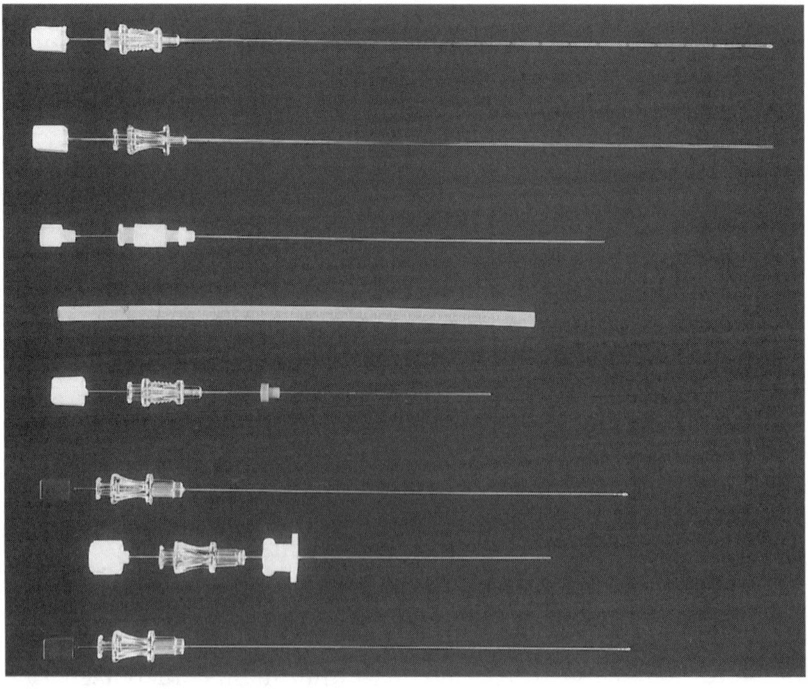

FIG. 11-1. *From top to bottom:* Chiba needle, Franseen (crown) needle, Turner needle with calibrated plastic sheath, Menghini needle, and three-piece coaxial system.

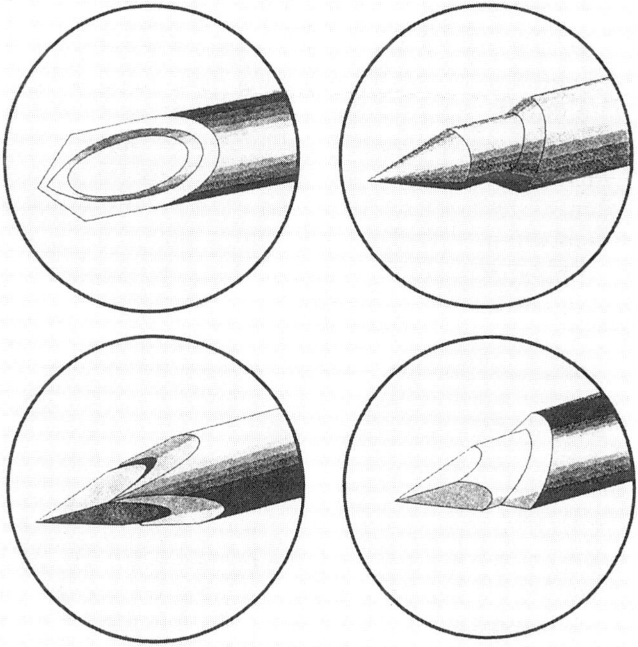

FIG. 11-2. *From top to bottom and clockwise from left to right:* Fine-needle aspiration tips. Chiba needle, Menghini needle, Franseen (crown) needle, and Turner needle.

markings on the needle itself, although a plastic outer sheath has markings at 1-cm intervals. This needle is particularly useful when a core biopsy of a very firm lesion is desirable.

Chiba Style Needle (Manan Medical Products)
This is a 20-cm-long, single-pass, 18-gauge needle marked at 1-cm intervals. The needle has a short beveled tip and an inner stylet that locks into place. The inner stylet does not protrude beyond the needle tip. Once the needle is in position within the nodule, patients are asked to hold their breaths. The stylet is withdrawn and a 20-cm^3 Luer lock syringe is attached to the needle hub. Suction is applied as the needle is moved back and forth within the nodule. The needle is then completely removed from the patient's chest.

Menghini Biopsy Needle (Manan Medical Products)
This is a 10-cm-long, single-pass, 20-gauge needle that has markings at 1-cm intervals. It has a short beveled edge and a

sharp inner stylet that protrudes about 0.4 cm beyond the tip of the needle. It is used identically to the Chiba style needle.

Wang Percutaneous Biopsy Needle (Mill-Rose Laboratories)
This 15-cm-long device consists of a 19-gauge outer needle and a 21-gauge inner needle, each with a beveled tip and inward-tapering cutting edge. A sharp-tipped stylet is inside the inner needle. The inner needle is connected by a short wire to a hub. When the hub is advanced and locked into place, the inner needle protrudes 0.5 cm beyond the tip of the outer needle. The outer needle has a side port for suction. The inner needle serves as a guide for the outer needle, which is advanced over the inner needle into the lesion. Once in the lesion, the stylet is removed, and a 20-mL Luer lock syringe filled with 3 to 5 cm^3 of saline solution is attached to the side port, either directly or using 20-in. intravenous extension tubing. The hub is unlocked and retracted. This withdraws the inner needle about 2 cm into the outer needle. The stylet is withdrawn, and suction is applied to the syringe. The outer needle is moved in and out of the nodule. With suction maintained, the entire needle is then removed from the patient's chest. The specimen is flushed from the needle tip using the saline and air in the syringe. A second pass may be necessary if a core of tissue has not been obtained.

Multiple-Pass Coaxial System Needles (Bauer Medical)
With this system, a 10-cm, 20-gauge, coaxial needle with 1-cm markings is inserted into the lesion. The needle is held firmly in position at the skin by turning a plastic lock that slides onto the needle itself. The inner stylet is removed, and a 15-cm, 22-gauge aspiration-biopsy needle is inserted through the coaxial guide. The inner stylet of this needle is withdrawn, and the specimen obtained after attaching a Luer lock syringe to the hub of the needle. This kit actually comes with two aspiration-biopsy needles, so that the second sample can be obtained while the first is being handled by the cytopathologist.

◆ Techniques

Before
Informed consent should include the indication for needle aspiration biopsy, a simple review of potential management options depending on the results of the procedure, and a description of potential complications and their treatment.

Appropriate laboratory personnel such as cytopathologists or bacteriologists are notified of the procedure and asked to "stand ready" to receive the specimen, either in the laboratory or in the procedure suite itself. Having laboratory personnel present to immediately examine the specimen in the procedure suite assures satisfactory sampling, reduces the need for multiple needle passes (reducing the chance for complications), and increases diagnostic yield.

The patient's chest radiographs (and CT scans, if available) are examined, and the chart is reviewed to note results of previous nondiagnostic interventions, detect bleeding abnormalities, and identify potential allergies to local anesthetics (lidocaine), skin degerming agents, or tape. Patients need to remain immobile throughout the procedure, which may last from 15 to 60 minutes. Therefore, most patients will benefit from administration of an anxiolytic such as midazolam. Some will also benefit from intramuscular injection of an analgesic. Atropine 0.5 to 1.2 mg by intramuscular injection can be given at least 30 minutes before the procedure to help prevent vasovagal reactions. In higher risk individuals, intravenous access is warranted. Patients need not be NPO ("nothing by mouth").

During

Procedures are most easily performed with patients in the supine or prone position depending on nodule location. Careful positioning is essential in order to locate the abnormality, evaluate its positional changes during inspiration and expiration, determine its proximity to the chest wall, visualize needle depth and direction, and select the best entry site out of the way of bony structures such as the scapula.

An assistant should stand by the patient to monitor vital signs, offer comfort to the patient with soothing words of reassurance, administer additional medication as needed, and keep the patient from moving. A pillow can be placed beneath the patient's head to improve comfort. Instruments for chest tube insertion should be readily available.

Careful examination of the anterior or posterior chest wall precedes selection of the target area. When the patient is lying supine, both arms are kept at his or her sides, pulling the shoulders back and expanding the anterior and lateral intercostal spaces. When the patient is lying prone, the arms and shoulders are raised so that hands are folded under his or her forehead. This pulls the scapulae outward and upward.

Under imaging guidance, the intrapulmonary abnormality is located and the appropriate skin projection noted using a radiopaque marker (a needle, a paper clip, or the tip of a metal hanger or piano wire will usually suffice). The site for needle insertion is marked using a sterile marking pen. If fluoroscopy is employed, the lesion is viewed in more than one plane to determine lesion depth. This will help guide needle insertion.

Skin disinfection is confined to the target area of needle aspiration. A wide preparation is unnecessary. Povidone-iodine solution should be applied to the skin using sterile gauze, then blotted dry. Local anesthesia is provided using 1% or 2% lidocaine injected through a 25-gauge needle. First, a large wheal is raised at the skin and subcutaneous tissues overlying the upper margin of the rib at the planned needle insertion site. Using a 2-in., 22-gauge needle and a 3-cm^3 syringe, additional lidocaine is injected through the wheal perpendicularly into the subcutaneous and intercostal tissues, with care taken to remain above the superior margin of the underlying rib. The parietal pleura is infiltrated, but insertion of the needle into the lung parenchyma is avoided. The needle is maintained perpendicular to the chest wall (it can be grasped with long ring forceps) while imaging is performed to assure that the needle is being inserted in the direction of the intrapulmonary lesion.

Once these tissues are infiltrated, a small stab incision using a no. 11 scalpel is made to facilitate insertion of the aspiration-biopsy needle through the skin. This needle is inserted a short distance into the chest wall. Intermittent imaging studies, such as fluoroscopy in the frontal projection, are used to verify that the needle is moving toward the lesion and that the needle tip is centered over the lesion. Again, the needle can be held in position using long ring forceps while imaging studies are obtained. This avoids irradiating the operator's hands. The tip of the needle is aligned with the rib interspace and the intrapulmonary nodule while the patient is asked to take slow, shallow breaths; patients can also be instructed to intermittently hold their breath. If an adjustment is necessary, the needle should be partially withdrawn and redirected. Simply tilting the needle tip toward the lesion without withdrawing the needle is rarely successful; in fact, it increases the chance of tearing through visceral pleura.

Under direct imaging guidance, the needle is inserted gradually through lung parenchyma until it enters the lesion. It may be necessary to stop needle advancement several times for imaging purposes in order to assure that the needle is moving in the correct direction (Fig. 11-3). As the needle enters the nodule, a change in consistency is often felt; many nodules are firm or rubbery. Holding the needle again with a long ring forceps, imaging will verify that the needle tip is well into the nodule. Often, the nodule can be seen to move laterally left and right under fluoro-

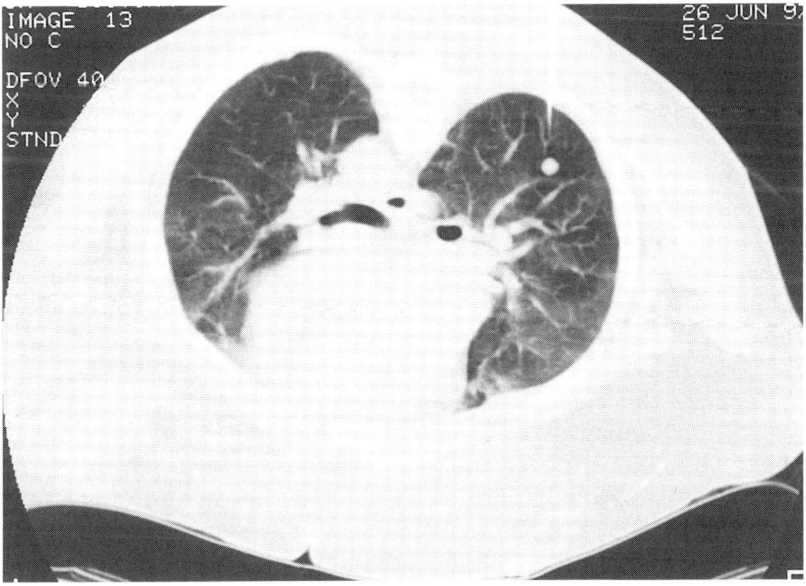

FIG. 11-3. Computed tomography scan of small peripheral nodule and percutaneous fine-needle aspiration. Note stepwise progression with imaging revealing that needle is moving in the direction of the nodule. Diagnosis was metastatic adenocarcinoma.

scopic guidance as the needle is gently pushed laterally back and forth. The inner stylet or needle guide is removed, a Luer lock syringe is attached at the proximal end of the needle, and the cytology or histopathology specimen is obtained.

Suction is applied by withdrawing the needle plunger so that material obtained from the nodule is aspirated into the tip of the needle, not up into the hub of the syringe. For this reason, aspiration is best accomplished by simply using an empty 20-mL plastic or glass syringe attached to the proximal hub of the needle. Suction is applied once the needle is inside the nodule and while gently moving the needle in and out of the lesion. Additional passes are performed as needed until enough material is obtained for diagnostic studies.

After

After the needle has been removed from the patient, the syringe is removed from the needle, and 5 to 10 mL of air is aspirated into the syringe, which is reattached to the needle. The material contained in the tip of the needle is then injected onto slides or into preservative for cytology and microbiology. If a core biopsy was obtained, it is injected into a container with 10% formalin solution for histologic examination.

Immediately upon completion of the procedure, fluoroscopy or CT imaging is warranted to verify the absence of pneumothorax. Frontal fluoroscopic imaging may not always visualize a small pneumothorax when patients are in the supine or prone position. If patients are stable and there is no evidence of pneumothorax on immediate fluoroscopic or CT imaging, the skin is cleaned of blood or povidone-iodine. A compressive sterile dressing is applied for at least 24 hours. Two-view chest radiographs (posteroanterior and lateral) are warranted within 1 to 4 hours after the procedure to detect a procedure-related pneumothorax.

Because the risk of pneumothorax is high after fine-needle aspiration biopsy of pulmonary nodules, patients are usually observed in a postprocedure area for several hours before returning to the ward or being discharged. In the case of outpatient procedures, patients are instructed to have someone with them for at least the first 24 hours after the procedure, and to immediately call or return to the hospital in case of hemoptysis, dizziness, or shortness of breath.

The ideal fine-needle aspiration biopsy procedure note should include (1) the indication for needle aspiration or biopsy (e.g., patient with a 2-cm unilateral right-sided solitary pulmonary nodule and significant smoking history); (2) the results of previous diagnostic and nondiagnostic interventions; (3) a description of the procedure, including the needle used, the insertion site (e.g., three finger breadths above the right nipple) and which intercostal space and hemithorax were accessed; (4) the number of needle passes and whether specimens were obtained for cytology, histopathology, and microbiology; (5) imaging modality employed (fluoroscopy or CT); (6) the patient's tolerance of the procedure and medications required; (7) whether any adverse events occurred; and (8) the results of postprocedure imaging studies including the chest radiograph.

▼ Complications

- Pneumothorax related to introduction of a small amount of air during the procedure should be expected in less than 10% of instances. This is best avoided by using breath-holding techniques during removal and insertion of inner stylets and needle biopsy guides. Treatment is usually not necessary.
- Pneumothorax related to laceration of lung parenchyma and visceral pleural tears can be expected in up to 30% of

cases when intrapulmonary nodules are sampled. The risk of pneumothorax is greater than after bronchoscopic lung biopsy and may be increased in patients with lesions located deep within the lung parenchyma. Most operators believe that risk is also increased in patients with bullous emphysema and other forms of obstructive lung disease, although some debate persists on this issue. Pneumothorax will usually cause symptoms such as cough, pleuritic chest discomfort, or dyspnea. Symptoms, or a pneumothorax greater than 10% in size, should prompt immediate small-bore chest tube insertion to relieve symptoms and reexpand the lung.

- Hemoptysis occurs in less than 5% of fine-needle aspirations and biopsies. It is usually transient and may be related to needle size. Some patients may expectorate blood-tinged sputum during the procedure when blood from the biopsy site reaches the central airways. This occurs most frequently during biopsies of anterior segment, upper lobe lesions.
- Hemothorax can occur from inadvertent laceration of intercostal vessels or lung parenchyma. Careful technique helps avoid this complication. Remember that the internal mammary artery lies approximately 2 cm lateral to the sternal border.
- Vasovagal reactions occur infrequently and can probably be avoided almost altogether by keeping this procedure anxiety- and pain-free.
- Contamination of the needle tract by infectious organisms is extremely rare and easily avoided by the use of proper sterile techniques.
- Arterial air embolism has been described in less than 0.1% of cases, but may occur when large biopsy needles are used and air enters through the needle directly or as a result of iatrogenic formation of a bronchovenous or bronchoalveolovenous fistula. Symptoms suggestive of cardiovascular collapse should prompt immediate placement into the Trendelenberg position, administration of 100% oxygen, and transfer to a hyperbaric chamber to promote resorption of air bubbles.

☆ Clinical Pearls

- To assure a satisfactory diagnostic yield, a cytopathologist should be present during the procedure to immediately examine the material obtained.

- In patients with abundant subcutaneous tissue or muscle, a 14-gauge angiocatheter can be used as a conduit for the smaller gauge, more flexible aspiration-biopsy needle.
- Breath holding techniques are difficult for many patients. Often it is easier to synchronize needle insertion with the patient's respiratory movements.
- When using fluoroscopy, most procedures can be satisfactorily performed using only frontal projections as long as the tip of the needle is kept centered over the lesion. Occasionally, a simple oblique view will indicate that the nodule is being pushed away from the needle as it is being entered.
- In nodules with potentially necrotic centers, it is often desirable to sample the periphery of the nodule as well.
- Needle insertion paths from the skin to the intrapulmonary nodule should be kept perpendicular to the chest wall.

Heard on the Wards

Question: How do I know whether to use fluoroscopic or computed tomography guidance?

Answer: Most nodules can be accessed using fluoroscopic guidance. Fluoroscopy is usually more readily available and less expensive than CT. Some nodules, however, are not readily visible, so CT imaging is warranted in these. Patients need to be more cooperative in their control of breathing when CT is used, and they must be able to lie still in the scanner during the procedure.

Question: When should I be thinking of doing fine-needle aspiration instead of bronchoscopic lung biopsy?

Answer: Most investigators agree that fine-needle aspiration should be considered instead of bronchoscopic lung biopsy in patients with small (less than 2 cm) pulmonary nodules, or when nodules are peripheral or abutting the chest wall. The diagnostic yield of bronchoscopic lung biopsy in these cases is well below 50%. Diagnostic yield of fine-needle aspiration in cases where cancer or granulomatous disease such as tuberculosis, coccidioidomycosis, cryptococcosis, and histoplasmosis is present is probably in the 60% to 80% range. However, the risk of pneumothorax is greater for fine-needle aspiration procedures (up to 30%) than it is for bronchoscopic lung biopsy (less than 5%).

Question: Are there indications for fine-needle aspiration biopsy other than pulmonary nodules?

Answer: Fine-needle aspiration biopsy is indicated for diagnosis of rib lesions, as well as tumors and infections involving the soft tissues of the chest wall. In these cases, care is taken to avoid entering the pleural space and lung. Mediastinal and perihilar abnormalities can also be sampled, but most oncologists prefer larger tissue samples for definitive diagnosis of tumor and lymphoma.

Question: What are the advantages and disadvantages of single-pass and multiple-pass coaxial needle systems?

Answer: The single-pass needle makes a very small hole in the pleura, thereby minimizing pleural trauma and risk for pneumothorax. However, because the needle is withdrawn entirely to process each specimen and then reinserted, the procedure may take longer and the nodule may not be properly accessed on each successive pass. The multiple-pass coaxial needle systems require a larger bore needle, so that risk of pneumothorax is possibly greater. Once inside the lesion, however, the needle guide is not withdrawn and multiple samples are quickly processed without difficulty (provided the patient does not move).

✔ Procedural Guidelines: Fine-Needle Aspiration Biopsy

History and physical examination
Review chest radiographs and CT scans
Assess coagulation profile and lung function
Review results of previous studies
Select fluoroscopic or CT guidance.

↓

Prepare patient and equipment

← Prepare instrument tray and specimen containers
Select appropriate needle
Have cytopathologist available

→ Position patient
Localize nodule
Monitor vital signs

↓

Perform fine needle aspiration biopsy

Tissue analysis
Multiple passes only if required by cytopathologist.
Move needle in and out of lesion while maintaining suction.
Flush needle and inject specimen into preservative for cytology and into sterile container for microbiology.

Helpful hints
Abundant local anesthesia.
Sedation and analgesia often helpful.
Ascertain needle depth to nodule.
Stepwise insertion under imaging guidance.
Synchronize needle insertion with patient's breathing pattern.

Recovery
Always obtain procedure chest radiograph.
Verify absence of pneumothorax.
Follow-up in case of hemoptysis, dyspnea, cough, or chest pain.

Recommended Reading

Aberle DR, Gamsu G, Golden JA. Fatal systemic arterial air embolism following lung needle aspiration. Radiology 1987; 165:351–353.

Fatalities can occur, albeit very rarely.

Anderson CL, Acevedo Crespo JC, Lie TH. Risk of pneumothorax not increased by obstructive lung disease in percutaneous needle biopsy. Chest 1994;105:1705–1708.

Questions previous reports suggesting a linear correlation between degree of obstructive ventilatory impairment and risk of pneumothorax.

Miller KS, Fish GD, Stanley JH, Schabel SI. Prediction of pneumothorax rate in percutaneous needle aspiration of the lung. Chest 1988;93:742–745.

Fivefold increase in incidence of pneumothorax in patients with obstructive lung disease compared to normals.

Mueller PR, van Sonnenberg E. Interventional radiology in the chest and abdomen. N Engl J Med 1990;322:1364–1375.

A review of interventional radiology techniques by two leaders in the field.

Wang KP, Gonullu U, Baker R. Bronchoscopy needle aspiration versus transthoracic needle aspiration in the diagnosis of pulmonary lesions. J Bronchol 1994;1:199–204.

Diagnostic yield of transthoracic fine-needle aspiration was 70% among 105 patients who had previously nondiagnostic bronchoscopic lung biopsy.

12. CLOSED-TUBE THORACOSTOMY USING SMALL-BORE CHEST TUBES

✣ Definition

Percutaneous insertion of a small-caliber tube through an intercostal space into the pleural cavity to drain fluid or air and to reexpand the lung.

❍ Indications

- Iatrogenic pneumothorax, initial spontaneous pneumothorax, and loculated pneumothorax.
- Loculated pleural effusions, complicated parapneumonic effusions, and empyema.
- Most appropriate when pleural ultrasonography, fluoroscopy, or computed tomography scans document small, loculated pleural collections that are not easily accessible using non-image-guided techniques and do not require manual debridement of fibrinous adhesions.

● Contraindications

- Substantial pleuropulmonary adhesions making instrumental access to the pleural space difficult and unsafe.
- Uncorrected coagulopathy.
- Lack of informed consent or patient cooperation.

❖ Equipment

Argyle-Turkel Safety Pneumothorax Catheter (Sherwood, Davis, and Geck)

This is a 9-cm-long, 8-Fr, polyurethane catheter-over-needle device attached to a spring-loaded safety canal that indicates loss of resistance of tissue as the catheter penetrates through parietal pleura, thereby avoiding "sharps" in the pleural cavity. The short, soft catheter makes kinking at the entrance site, as well as its use in muscular or obese individuals, problematic (Fig. 12-1).

Tru-Close Thoracic Vent (Sherwood, Davis, and Geck)

This is a 10-cm-long, 13-Fr, polyurethane catheter with an outer diameter of 4.2 mm. The catheter is incorporated into a small box containing a one-way valve, red-signal diaphragm, and adhesive patch for fixation to the skin. The catheter rarely kinks but is too short for use in obese patients.

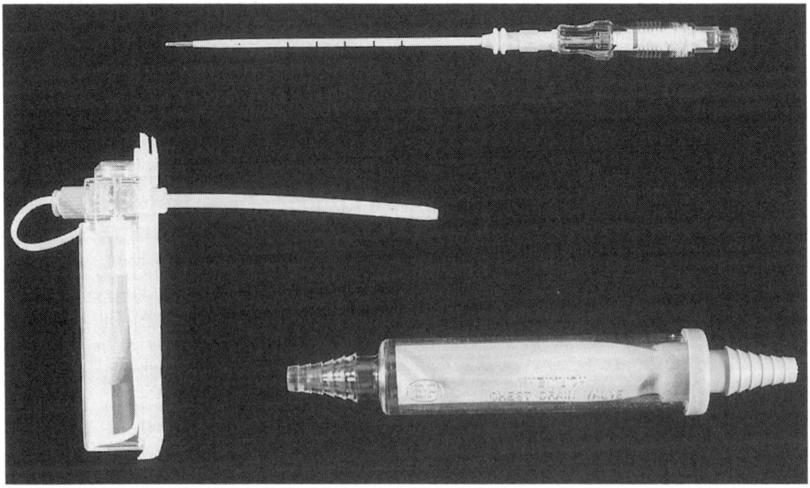

FIG. 12-1. Argyle-Turkel safety chest drainage catheter *(top)*, Tru-Close thoracic vent *(middle)*, and one-way Heimlich valve *(bottom)*.

Arrow Pneumothorax Set (Arrow International)
This is a 16-cm-long, 8-Fr, catheter-over-needle device made of polyurethane. Kinking occurs easily at the entrance site because the catheter becomes softer at body temperature. The set includes a one-way valve (Fig. 12-2).

Arrow Cavity Drainage Catheters (Arrow International)
These radiopaque polyurethane catheters come in 23-cm-long, 14-Fr diameters with straight or curved "pigtail" J-tip distal extremities and a proximal hub that includes a Luer lock connection. It is inserted over an inner dilator using the Seldinger technique. All components have centimeter markings.

Cook Percutaneous Chest Tube Sets (Cook Critical Care)
These catheter-over-needle devices come as 29-cm-long, rigid 9-Fr Teflon catheters and 10-Fr polyurethane catheters. Catheters can be attached to suction tubing prior to insertion into the pleural space. The sharp tip of the inner trocar extends past the catheter tip and should be quickly withdrawn into the inner trocar and catheter once the tube is inside the pleural space in order to avoid inadvertent puncture of lung parenchyma. Kits come with a one-way valve (Fig. 12-3).

Van Sonnenberg Sump Catheters (Medi-tech Boston Scientific)
Inserted either by direct trocar puncture or by the Seldinger technique, these soft radiopaque Percuflex catheters come in 30- to 35-

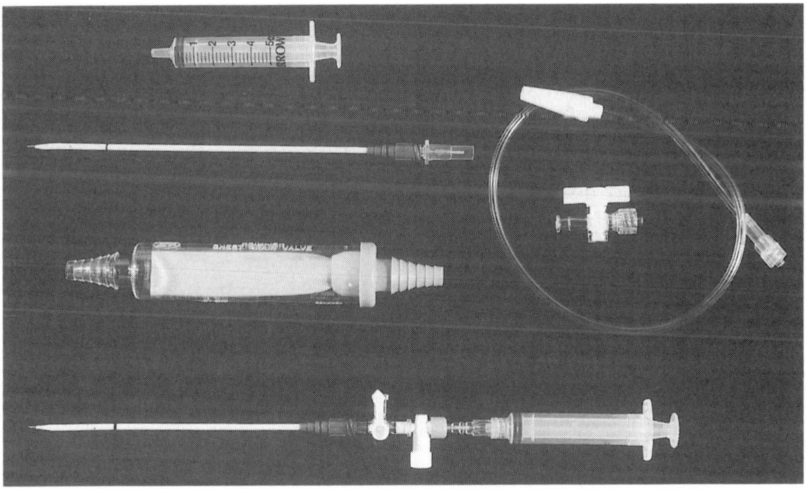

FIG. 12-2. Arrow percutaneous 8-Fr pneumothorax *(top)* and thoracentesis catheter with stopcocks *(bottom)*. Kits come with one-way Heimlich valve and extension tubing.

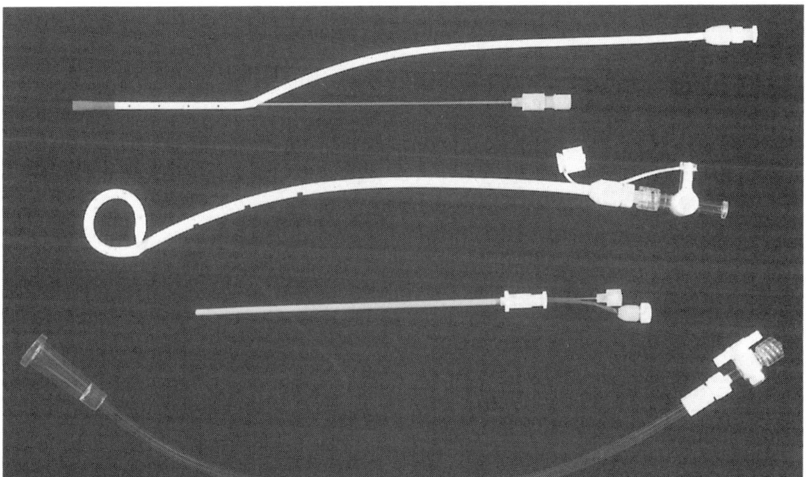

FIG. 12-3. Cook TPT *(top)* and Wayne pigtail *(middle)* pneumothorax sets with inner trocars and extension tubing *(bottom)* for connections to one-way Heimlich valves or collection bag.

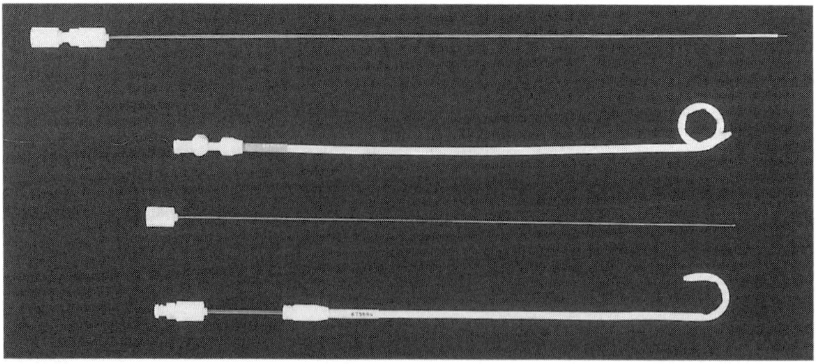

FIG. 12-4. Medi-tech Van Sonnenberg percutaneous chest drainage systems: 12-Fr pigtail *(top)* and J tube *(bottom)* with insertion trocars.

cm lengths in sizes 12 to 16 Fr. They are firm enough to not be compressed by the ribs. The distal extremity can be J-tip or locked into a pigtail after insertion by using a monofilament suture that extends from the catheter tip to the proximal hub, thereby preventing inadvertent withdrawal from the pleural space (Fig. 12-4).

Small-Bore Chest Tube Insertion Techniques

Before

Each of the above-described chest tube kits comes with well-written instructions for insertion using either catheter-over-needle or catheter-over-guidewire techniques. Preparation and local anesthesia of the selected target site are done as for thoracentesis. Before inserting the chest tube it is wise to confirm the presence of air or fluid in the pleural space using a 22-gauge needle mounted on a 20-cm^3 syringe and inserted through the planned site of incision.

During

A small stab incision is made using a no. 11 scalpel. The needle–syringe ensemble is advanced over the rib. Insertion into the

FIG. 12-5. Catheter over guidewire (Seldinger) technique of small-bore chest tube insertion. The pleural space is accessed **(a).** The guidewire is thread through the needle **(b).** The dilator is thread over the guidewire, then revmoved **(c)**. The chest tube is thread over the guidewire **(d)**. The guidewire is removed, leaving the chest tube in position. The chest tube will be secured using a simple stitch tied down onto the chest tube using a surgeon's knot **(e)**.

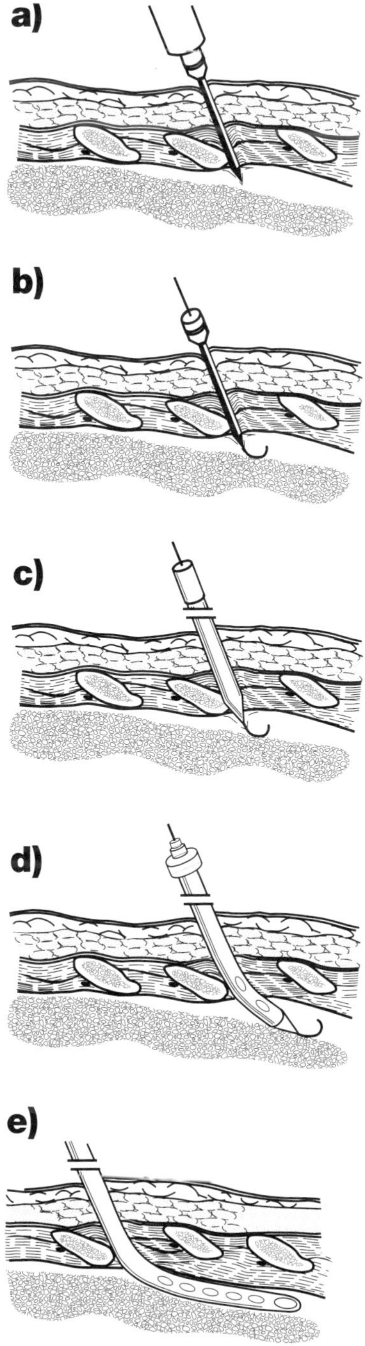
a)
b)
c)
d)
e)

pleural space is confirmed by aspiration of air or fluid. The catheter is threaded over the needle, with care taken not to withdraw the needle during catheter insertion. Once the catheter is sufficiently in the pleural space, the needle is withdrawn and the catheter connected to the thoracic drainage device or one-way valve. The catheter-over-guidewire (Seldinger) technique requires gradual dilatation of the insertion tract. Access to the pleural space is identical to that described earlier, although tunneling the catheter obliquely beneath the skin along a distance of at least one intercostal space helps maintain tube stability. A guidewire is then inserted through the needle as the needle is withdrawn. A small stab incision widens the tract immediately adjacent to the wire. Dilators of gradually increasing size are threaded over the wire and through the intercostal tissues and parietal pleura. The chest tube is similarly threaded over the guidewire until it is in its appropriate position within the pleural space (Fig. 12-5). A single zero-silk suture placed adjacent to the tube, or a Molnar retention disk, is used to secure the tube in position, after which a transparent dressing is placed over the insertion site.

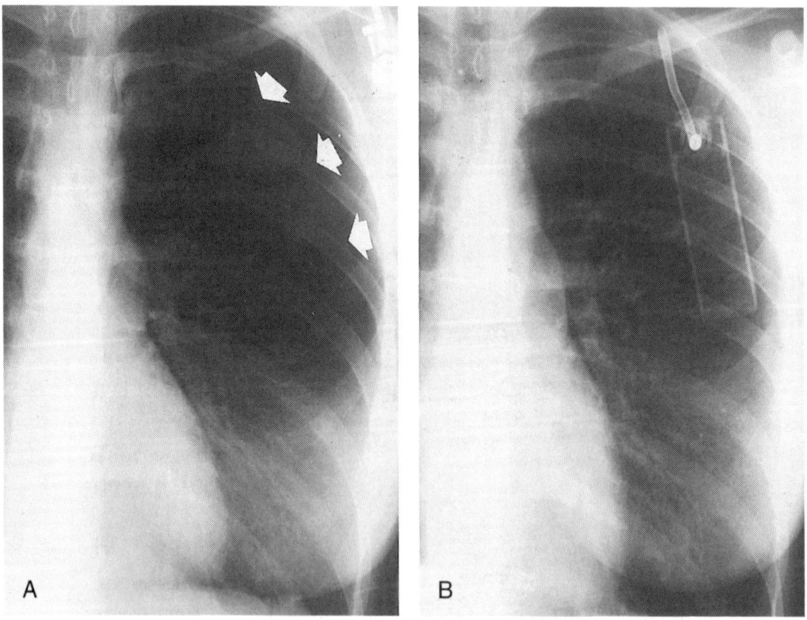

FIG. 12-6. Chest radiographs of a patient with iatrogenic pneumothorax following bronchoscopic lung biopsy **(A)**. Insertion of a Tru-Close thoracic vent through the second intercostal space of the left anterior hemithorax resulted in complete lung reexpansion **(B)**.

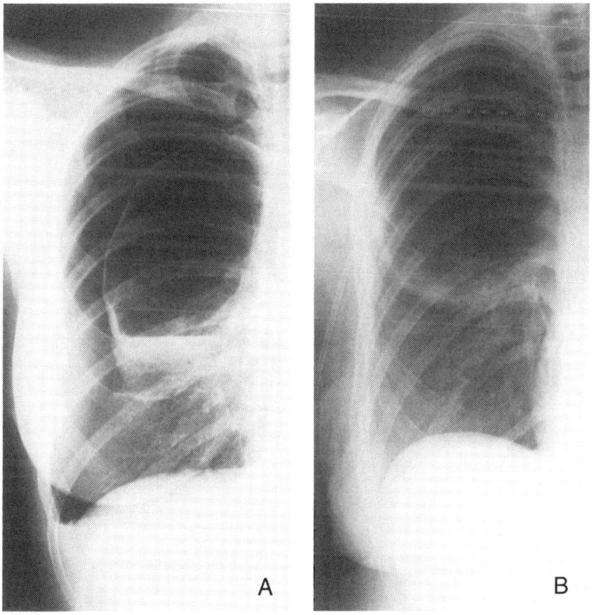

FIG. 12-7. Chest radiographs of a recurrent spontaneous pneumothorax in a young woman with a large unilateral right-sided bulla. Note the small effusion collected in the costophrenic angle, and the thickened margins of the partially collapsed bulla and small air-fluid level **(A)**. The lung has reexpanded after insertion of a small-bore Cook TPT chest tube. The bulla is clearly visible occupying more than half of the hemithorax. The chest tube is a too high apically and medially, causing mild patient discomfort **(B)**. It will be pulled back about 2 cm.

After

The chest tube is attached to either a one-way valve or the negative suction device. Care is taken to avoid excessive traction on the small tube, which may cause pain, kinking, or even inadvertent removal of the tube from the pleural cavity. A posteroanterior or portable chest radiograph is obtained to assure chest tube position and lung reexpansion (Figs. 12-6 and 12-7).

The ideal small-bore chest tube insertion note should include (1) the indication for the procedure; (2) the amount and type of premedication or sedation; (3) the site of insertion (e.g., 2nd intercostal space along the midclavicular line of the left anterior chest); (4) a description of the technique and chest tube used (e.g., 8-Fr pigtail catheter using the Seldinger technique); (5) the tube's direction and final position (e.g., the tube was directed cephalad and anteriorly toward the apex of the left hemithorax); (6) a description of air or fluid evacuated into the thoracic drainage device; (7) the patient's tolerance of the procedure and a description of any adverse events; (8) results of the postprocedure chest radiograph verifying chest tube position and resultant evacuation of pleural fluid or air and lung reexpansion.

▼ Complications

- Excessive chest wall discomfort is seen less frequently than after large-tube insertion. A large cutaneous wheal should be raised, and a small stab incision makes insertion of the trocar through the skin easier.
- Shoulder pain is avoided by not directing the distal tip of the chest tube too high in the apex of the hemithorax. If the distal tip is above the clavicle on the chest radiograph, it can be pulled back slightly.
- Inadvertent laceration of intercostal vessels is easily avoided by inserting tubes directly above the superior margin of the underlying rib.
- Chest tube malfunction is usually the result of kinking or obstruction from fluid, fibrin, or blood. The absence of fluctuation in the water seal chamber of the thoracic drainage device should prompt syringe aspiration of the chest tube and, if necessary, flushing of the chest tube with sterile saline or 100,000 to 250,000 U/mL of urokinase to reestablish patency.
- Inadvertent laceration of the lung is avoided by ascertaining that sufficient pleural fluid or air is present in the pleural space at the site of insertion, and by removing sharp trocars the moment the pleural cavity is entered. If necessary, a small pneumothorax can be created and the lung allowed to collapse away from the chest wall at the time of the incision or trocar insertion.
- Subcutaneous emphysema is rare unless proximal side holes of the chest tube are left within extrapleural tissues.
- Extrapleural insertion should be avoided by use of proper localization and insertion techniques.

☆ Clinical Pearls

- Exploratory thoracentesis should be attempted at the projected site of chest tube insertion to confirm the presence of air or fluid.

- Any misconnections (adapters, Luer locks) can cause an air leak.
- If air leaks are prolonged and/or continuous, inadvertent intraparenchymal insertion of the chest tube should be considered.
- In order to avoid lung puncture, stiff dilators and trocars should not be firmly pushed into the pleural cavity.
- If malpositioned, tubes can be pulled back, but they should not be advanced because of the risk of lung injury or pleural space contamination.

Heard on the Wards

Question: What if I suspect adhesions between the lung and chest wall?

Answer: A pneumothorax can be induced using the "drop technique." A 20-gauge needle is inserted through the skin at the incision site. The needle is first filled to the hub with saline solution. As the needle enters the pleural space, the negative intrapleural pressure prompts aspiration of the saline solution, which drops into the pleural space. As the patient takes a few breaths, additional air enters the pleural cavity, causing the lung to collapse away from the chest wall.

Question: How do I verify intrapleural tube insertion?

Answer: Intrapleural insertion is confirmed by aspirating air or fluid through the chest tube before it is fixed into place and before connecting it to the thoracic drainage device. Condensation may be noted in the chest tube during respiration. After connecting the tube to the drainage device, fluctuation should be noted in the water seal chamber with the patient off suction.

Question: Is there a rule of thumb for selecting chest tube size?

Answer: Tubes smaller than 20 Fr usually suffice for iatrogenic pneumothoraces where air leaks are small and are seldom associated with pleural fluid drainage. Small tubes may also be warranted in selected cases of loculated effusions or to rapidly drain a large effusion. Larger tubes (28 Fr and above) are usually used in patients with secondary pneumothoraces from trauma or rupture of bullae, to enhance lung reexpansion after thoracoscopy or lung resection, to drain large effusions, blood, or pus from the pleural space, and for pleurodesis.

✔ Procedural Guidelines: Small-Bore Chest Tube Insertion

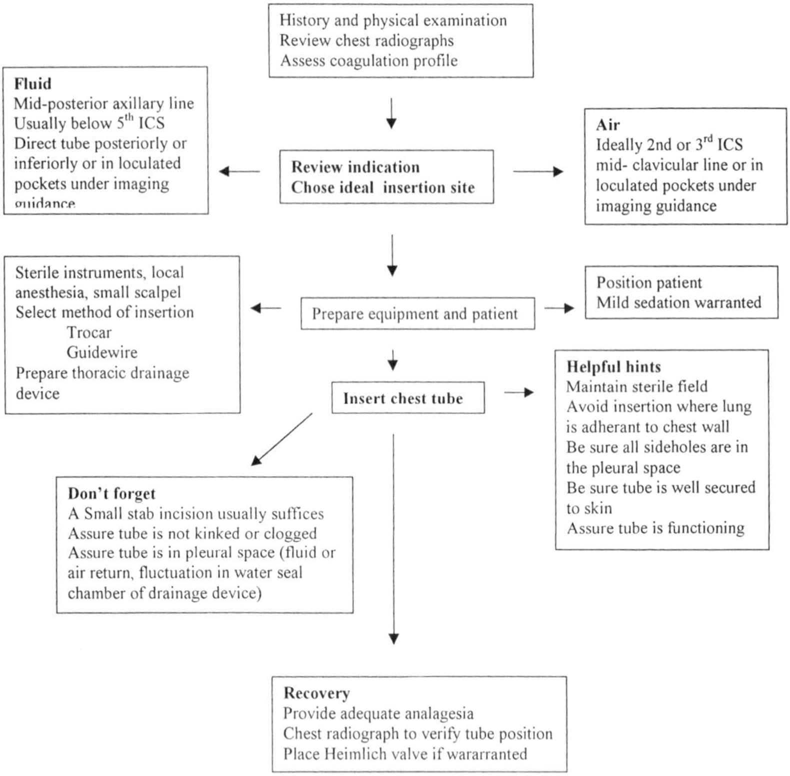

Recommended Reading

Bonnet RB, Aghili S. Small caliber tube thoracostomy. J Bronchol 1996;3:311–315.

A description of the author's technique.

Casola B, van Sonnenberg E, Keightley A, Ho M, Wither C, Lee AS. Pneumothoraces: radiologic treatment with small catheters. Radiology 1988;166:89–91.

A series of 30 patients (15 under tension) for which 28 were successfully treated using 7- to 9.4-Fr chest tubes.

Martin T, Fontana G, Olak J, Ferguson M. Use of a pleural catheter for the management of simple pneumothorax. Chest 1996;110:1169–1172.

The thoracic vent was successful in resolving 85% of 84 spontaneous or iatrogenic pneumothoraces studied. Average duration of catheter insertion was 3 days.

Samelson SL, Goldberg EM, Ferguson MK. The thoracic vent: clinical experience with a new device for treating simple pneumothorax. Chest 1991;100:880–882.
Easy to insert, particularly in the emergency room setting.
Ulmer JL, Choplin RH, Reed JC. Image-guided catheter drainage of the infected pleural space. J Thorac Imaging 1991;6:65–73.
A review article that also describes irrigation techniques.

13. CLOSED-TUBE THORACOSTOMY USING LARGE-BORE CHEST TUBES

✤ Definition

Insertion of a large-caliber chest tube into the pleural cavity through a 1- to 2-in. incision made along an intercostal space to evacuate fluid and air, and to reexpand the lung.

❍ Indications

- Empyema, hemothorax, abundant pleural effusions.
- Spontaneous, secondary, or iatrogenic pneumothorax, particularly if prolonged air leak is suspected.
- For pleurodesis of recurrent malignant or benign pleural effusions.

● Contraindications

- Uncorrected coagulopathy, unless absolutely necessary.
- Lack of informed consent or patient cooperation.

✤ Equipment

Many hospitals have readily available large-bore **chest tube insertion trays** available on a portable cart. These should include a disposable razor, disinfectant detergent (povidone-iodine scrub), sterile gauze, sterile towels, at least four towel clips, 1% lidocaine, a 1-cm^3 syringe and 25-gauge needle for cutaneous anesthesia, a 20-cm^3 syringe and 22-gauge needle for

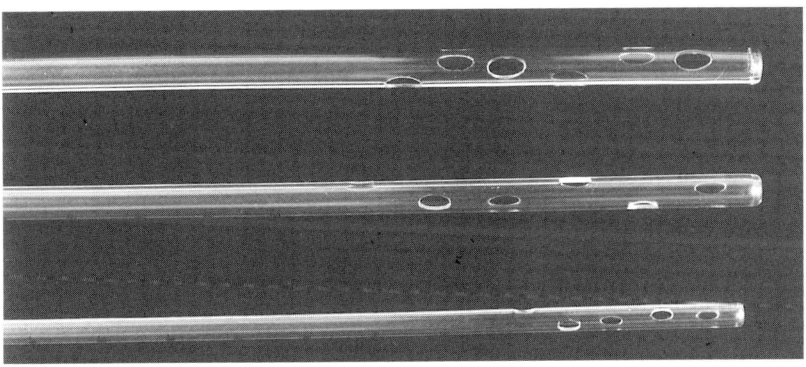

FIG. 13-1. Argyle chest tubes sizes 32 Fr, 28 Fr, and 20 Fr *(top to bottom)*. Notice how the sentinel holes farthest from the distal extremity of each tube are cut on the radiopaque line.

intercostal and parietal pleura anesthesia, three hemostats with small tips (used for blunt dissection of the intercostal tissues and to hold sutures), two large chest tube clamps with large blunt tips (used to hold the distal extremity of the chest tube during insertion and to clamp the tube once inserted), a needle driver and forceps, curved scissors, a no. 11 scalpel, three zero-silk sutures for skin closure and to secure the chest tube, straight silicone chest tubes sizes 28 to 36 Fr, tincture of benzoin, and 2-in. adhesive tape (Fig. 13-1).

Large-Bore Chest Tube Insertion Techniques

Before

Patients are satisfactorily sedated using combinations of narcotics, midazolam, or hydroxyzine. If necessary, supplemental oxygen can be administered during chest tube insertion. Any coagulopathy should be corrected, if possible, by temporarily withholding anticoagulation medication, or by reversing active drugs with vitamin K or fresh-frozen plasma. Informed consent should be obtained but may not be possible in life-threatening emergency situations.

Although bedside chest tube insertion is possible, a specially equipped **procedure room** is preferable because increased **sterility** of the procedure is enhanced, nursing personnel are available, and adverse events are more easily controlled. External cannulas or tube-over-trocar techniques for large-bore chest tube insertion are blind techniques that increase the risk of laceration of intrathoracic or intraabdominal organs. If using a trocar or sequential dilatation and Seldinger procedure, such as with the Thal-Quick chest tube set, careful attention must be paid to technique (Fig. 13-2). These polyvinyl chloride tubes are available in 28- to 41-cm lengths and come in sizes 8 to 36 Fr (Cook Inc.). An **exploratory thoracentesis** is essential to confirm the presence of air or fluid at the insertion site, the trocar should be firmly grasped during insertion so that it cannot penetrate more than 3 cm into the pleural cavity, and the trocar should be partially withdrawn prior to advancing the chest tube once it is a few centimeters into the pleural space,

Most large-bore chest tubes can be safely inserted through the **5th intercostal space** on the midaxillary line. In some patients with pneumothorax, however, the **2nd intercostal space** along the midclavicular line can be chosen. In this case, it is often necessary to shorten the chest tube by cutting a few inches off its distal extremity in order to avoid having side holes placed in the extrapleural tissues. If patients are extremely muscular, a lower

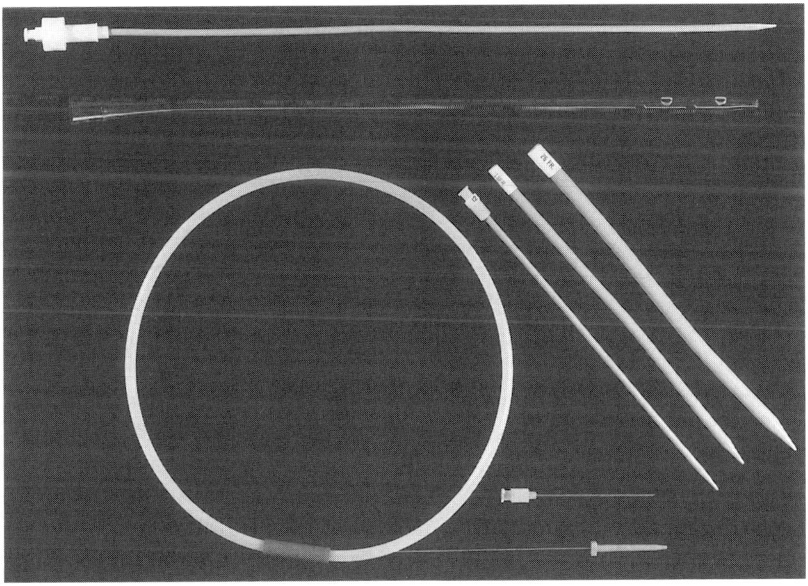

FIG. 13-2. Thal-Quick 24-Fr chest tube and dilators (Cook Inc.).

intercostal space may be chosen along the midaxillary line. Avoid placing tubes through the breast or thick muscular and adipose tissues because of the associated discomfort and risk of infection. In patients with adhesions and loculated air or fluid, the chest tube should be placed after an exploratory thoracentesis. Often, the tube can then be inserted at the site of thoracentesis. Tubes placed too posteriorly are uncomfortable and result in splinting, subsequent atelectasis, or lower respiratory tract infection.

During

With the patient supine, a rolled towel (also known as a bolster) is placed so that the target area is elevated about 20 degrees. Demerol (50 to 75 mg IM) and/or midazolam (1 to 5 mg IV) should be administered before starting. Body hair in the region of tube insertion and subsequent dressing is shaved using a disposable razor. A towel should also be placed beneath the patient to avoid soiling the bed with blood or detergent. If the patient is in a partial lateral decubitus position, the entire lateral chest is prepped with povidone-iodine. If the patient is supine, it is usually unnecessary to prep beyond the sternum. With care taken to not cover the patient's face, sterile towels are placed in rectangular fashion.

After raising a large subcutaneous wheal and anesthetizing the subcutaneous tissues, muscle planes, rib periosteum, and parietal pleura with generous (at least 30 cm^3) amounts of 1% lidocaine, a 2- to 4-cm transverse skin incision is made parallel to the rib along the intercostal space chosen for tube insertion or, if subcutaneous tunneling is desired, one intercostal space below.

Blunt dissection of the intercostal tissues is performed by spreading curved scissors or a blunt hemostat both parallel and perpendicular to the underlying muscle planes within the intercostal space. The intercostal muscles are separated, and the parietal pleura is gently penetrated over the superior margin of the 5th rib if using a lateral approach, or the 2nd rib if using an anterior approach. If necessary, additional local anesthetic can be injected directly onto the pleural surfaces. An index finger is gently inserted through the incision into the pleural space and adherent lung is pushed away from the chest wall. Rotating the fingertip in a firm but gentle circular fashion, adhesions are bluntly severed, allowing the lung to more readily collapse away from the chest wall. By enlarging the tract and assuring a free pleural space at the insertion site, the chance for extrapleural placement of the chest tube is minimized. The tip of the chest tube is grasped with a large, curved Kelly clamp and inserted through the incision into the pleural cavity. The clamp–chest tube ensemble can be inserted about 6 cm into the pleural cavity, after which the clamp is removed and the chest tube directed cephalad or caudal into its appropriate position (Fig. 13-3). The escape of air or fluid during tube insertion is not troublesome and there is no reason to inappropriately accelerate the insertion procedure. The chest tube hole most proximal to the operator (often referred to as the sentinel hole) should lie at least 2 cm inside the pleural cavity (Fig. 13-4). Once in place, the tube is connected to a thoracic drainage device and secured in position. If the tube is not secured with sutures before connecting to the thoracic drainage device, an assistant should hold the tube in place while it is being connected to keep it from being inadvertently pulled from the patient's chest.

Immediately before or after tube insertion, securing and resting zero-silk interrupted vertical mattress sutures should be placed through the incision site. Using this suture technique, equal bites of tissue are taken on each side of the skin incision. The deep bite closes subcutaneous tissues and muscles. The superficial bite provides an excellent approximation of skin edges. If unequal amounts of tissue are taken on either side of the incision, or if bites are of unequal depth on apposing sides of

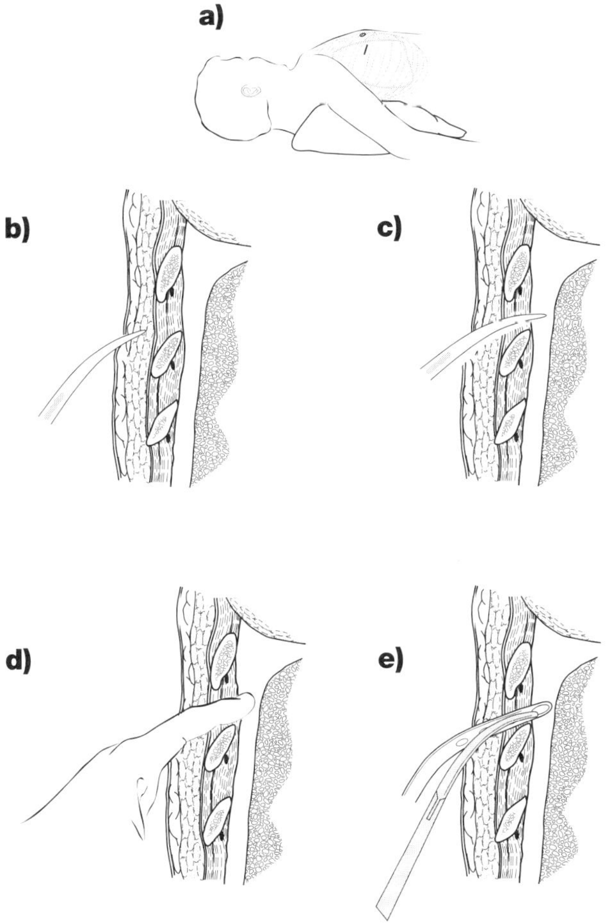

FIG. 13-3. Chest tube insertion techniques using blunt dissection. **A, B:** The 2- to 4-cm-long skin incision should be parallel to the intercostal space and made smoothly through the dermis, subcutaneous tissues, and fascia overlying the intercostal muscles. The intercostal muscle fibers are spread apart using the jaws of the scissors or a hemostat. By placing an index finger in the incision, the space between the muscle fibers is enlarged and the ribs are easily felt. **C:** Staying close to the upper margin of the lower rib, the intercostal fascia is sectioned, the intercostal muscles are spread further using the hemostat, and the parietal pleura is gently penetrated. **D:** An index finger will make the hole bigger and allow one to gently push the lung out of the way. **E:** After grasping the chest tube in the jaws of the clamp, guide it gently through the incision into the pleural space. Advance the tube well into the pleural space before releasing the clamp.

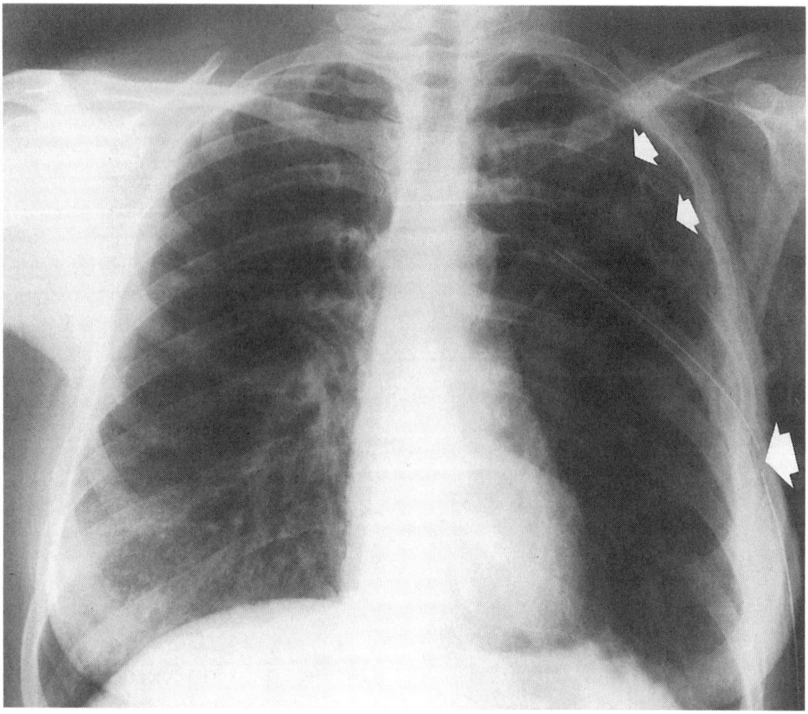

FIG. 13-4. Poorly placed large-bore chest tube in the major fissure of a patient with spontaneous pneumothorax. Also shows sentinel hole in extrapleural tissues *(large arrow)*, subcutaneous emphysema, and only partially reexpanded lung *(small arrows)*.

the incision, skin edges will overlap once the sutures are tied. First, a mattress suture is placed at each extremity of the incision. Then a mattress suture is placed through the middle of the incision for later use upon chest tube removal. Once the tube is in place, the lateral sutures are tied, closing each extremity of the incision. Each suture is then tied around the chest tube, securing it in place. A surgeon's knot is best used for this because it will not slide or loosen. To tie a surgeon's knot, make two turns of the suture about the first half-hitch and tighten the knot flatly on the chest tube. The second half-hitch can then be easily tied in the opposite direction and secured onto the double first half-hitch without risk of the first knot slipping. When the tube is removed, the resting suture placed across the middle of the incision is tied to the skin, approximating the edges and closing the incision entirely (Fig. 13-5). Another method is to use two purse-

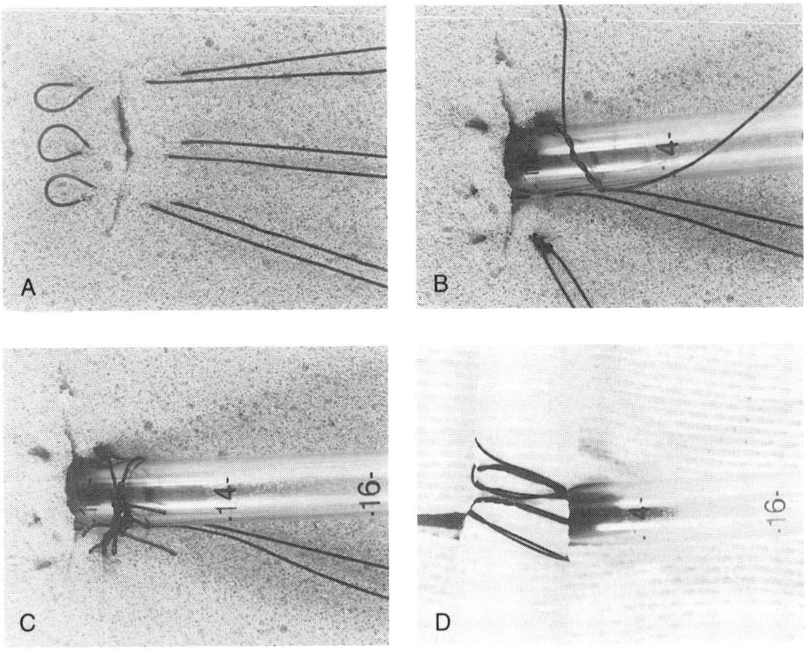

FIG. 13-5. Securing a chest tube into place using vertical interrupted mattress sutures. Healing is excellent even in the case of uneven margins. Three mattress sutures are placed through the incision **(A)**, the chest tube is inserted with care taken to not push the middle suture into the pleural cavity. Each lateral suture is tied to the skin, closing the lateral margins of the incision, then tied around the chest tube securing it into position using a surgeon's knot **(B, C)**. The middle suture, also referred to as the resting suture, is wrapped around a piece of gauze and tucked beneath the sterile dressing **(D)**. It will be tied down to close the central aspect of the incision at the time of chest tube removal.

string sutures that are easily tightened, closing the incision upon chest tube withdrawal (Fig. 13-6). If these sutures are tied too tightly, however, skin necrosis may occur.

After

A sterile and well cared for **dressing** is an important part of chest tube management. After chest tube insertion, the site should be cleaned of all povidone-iodine and thoroughly dried. Any body hair that may be covered by tape should be shaved. Split, sterile 4 × 4 gauze pads should be placed at the skin around the chest tube. The midincision **resting suture** can be

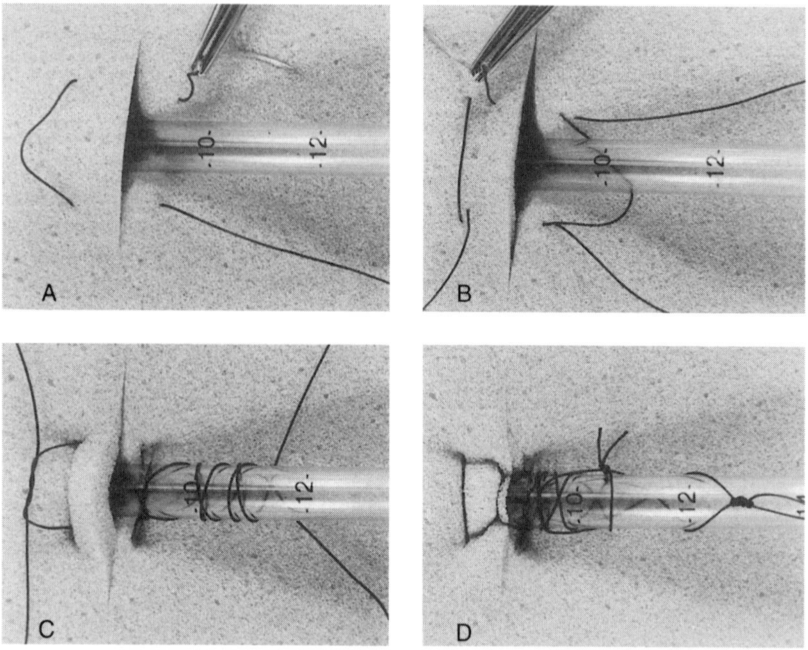

FIG. 13-6. Securing a chest tube using pursestring sutures. After chest tube insertion, two pursestring sutures are placed in opposite directions across the incision **(A, B)**. A flat, double knot tightens the skin around the chest tube **(C)**. Each suture is then wrapped and tied around the chest tube, leaving enough suture available so that each can be tied down and tightened to close the incision when the chest tube is removed **(D)**.

wrapped around a rolled 4 × 4 and inserted between the split pads. Two-inch tape placed from front to back over the lateral chest is used to secure the dressing. Silk tape is usually well tolerated and adheres well, yet it is easy to remove and does not leave too much sticky stuff on the skin. **Dressings** are routinely removed and inspected every 48 hours (or sooner if there is seepage from the incision site). A **banding gun** and serrated plastic Parham bands can be used to secure connections between the chest tube and suction tubing rather than taping these connections, which makes routine inspection laborious (Fig. 13-7).

The **ideal large-bore chest-tube insertion note** should include (1) the indication for the procedure; (2) the amount and type of premedication or sedation required; (3) the site of insertion (e.g., 5th intercostal space along the midaxillary line of the left lateral

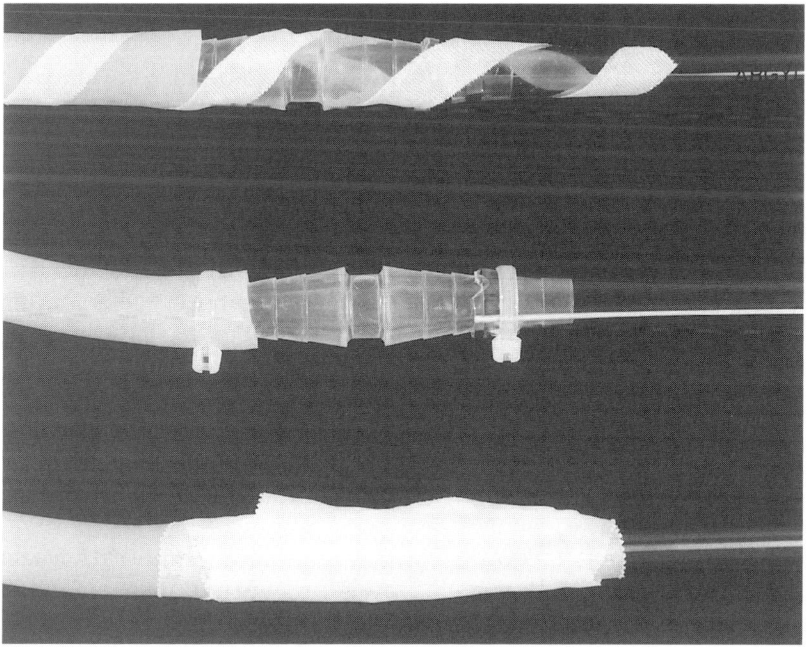

FIG. 13-7. Tube connections using a single strip of appropriately wrapped tape, Parham bands, and incorrectly wrapped tape *(top to bottom)*.

chest); (4) a description of the technique employed; (5) the state of the pleural cavity (e.g., firm adhesions were bluntly severed using an index finger through the incision site prior to chest tube insertion); (6) the size and type of chest tube inserted (e.g., 28-Fr straight silicone chest tube); (7) the tube's direction and final position (e.g., the tube was directed cephalad and anteriorly toward the apex of the left hemithorax); (8) a description of air or fluid evacuated during insertion; (9) the technique of closure of the incision site and securing of the chest tube; (10) the status of the thoracic drainage device (presence of fluid drainage, air leak, and fluctuation within the water seal chamber); and (11) the patient's tolerance of the procedure and a description of any adverse events.

▼ Complications

- Excessive chest wall discomfort can be avoided by the generous use of local anesthesia, intramuscular analgesia, and intravenous sedation; proper insertion technique; selection of a tube that fits easily through the incision site; and frequent dressing changes.

- Constant or pleuritic chest pain is avoided by not placing the chest tube too high in the axilla. Make sure that tubes are well secured and not easily pulled on or dangling from the bed.
- Inadvertent laceration of intercostal vessels should be avoided by never making deep, chopping scalpel incisions, by never introducing open scissors to dilate the incision site, and by inserting tubes directly above the superior margin of the underlying rib.
- Inadvertent laceration of the diaphragm, liver, spleen, or stomach can be avoided by paying careful attention to the insertion site, assuring that one is in the pleural space and not in the abdominal cavity, and by avoiding incision sites below the 6th or 7th intercostal space unless absolutely necessary.
- Inadvertent laceration of the lung or other intrathoracic organ should be avoided by gently introducing an index finger through the incision site into the pleural cavity to help separate the lung from the chest wall and to manually sever adhesions.
- Subcutaneous emphysema can occur if tubes are not firmly secured or if proximal side holes of the chest tube are within extrapleural tissues.
- Extrapleural insertion should be avoided by using proper localization and insertion techniques. If fluid or air is not removed and the thoracic drainage device does not appear to be functioning properly, tube malposition should be suspected.

☆ Clinical Pearls

- When in doubt, the skin incision should be ample enough to easily accommodate an index finger in the pleural cavity. The finger is used to gently push the expanded lung away from the chest wall and to break up adhesions around the chest tube entry site.
- If placing a large-bore chest tube high in the pleural space through a superior intercostal incision (2nd to 5th intercostal space), remember to measure the length of the chest cavity and to appropriately shorten the chest tube to avoid leaving side holes in the chest wall or outside the incision.
- If placing sutures before chest tube insertion, care must be taken to avoid pushing the sutures into the pleural space

with the tip of the tube or inadvertently securing the intrapleural part of the tube with a loop made in the underlying suture.

- Radiographically, the most proximal side hole (also called the sentinel side hole) can be seen because of a break in the radiopaque line that runs along the entire length of the large-bore chest tube. If an additional side hole must be cut in a tube, it should be placed along the radiopaque line. If holes are too numerous or too close together, the tube may kink.
- Tube caliber depends on indication. For empyema or hemothorax use 32- to 36-Fr tubes. For pleural effusion and possible pleurodesis, a 32-Fr tube usually suffices. For spontaneous pneumothorax, 28- to 32-Fr tubes work well, even when air leaks are large. For iatrogenic pneumothorax, a 20- to 28-Fr tube may be sufficient because air leaks are often smaller and generally resolve quickly.
- When dealing with a posterior loculated pleural effusion, especially in cases of empyema drainage, two approaches can be used. The chest tube can be inserted lateroposteriorly at a slight distance from the pleural collection and aimed toward the pleural collection. This is often more comfortable for the patient, who does not have to lie on the chest tube. The other approach is to insert the tube along the tract of the diagnostic thoracentesis. In this case, the incision is made "en face" of the loculated pocket of fluid and the chest tube is placed directly into the pleural collection. Don't forget to break down adhesions with your finger to enhance drainage of pus.

Heard on the Wards

Question: When placing a chest tube, what should I do if air enters the pleural space through my chest wall incision?

Answer: You have created an open pneumothorax. There is no need to rush because tension physiology is unlikely to occur as long as the open pneumothorax is maintained. Once accessed, both air or fluid can safely be allowed to gush out of the pleural cavity through the incision site while additional preparations for tube insertion, such as suture placement, are made. If necessary, the track into the pleural cavity can be maintained by insertion of the blunt extremity of a large clamp through the incision site.

Question: Is it really important for me to review the chest radiograph immediately after I've inserted a chest tube?

Answer: Yes. The proper functioning of this chest tube is your responsibility. This is your opportunity to verify tube placement and to feel a sense of accomplishment when you observe that the tube is positioned exactly where you want it. If, on the other hand, the tube is inappropriately positioned (e.g., high and anterior in a patient with empyema or a malignant pleural effusion), you may choose to immediately change it. If the tube is in the fissure, it may not need to be changed, but you can consider inserting another tube in a more appropriate position, or at least recognize that pleural drainage may not be as effective as you would have normally expected.

Question: Why not simply wrap tape around tubing connection sites?
Answer: Parham bands are much better than tape to secure tubing to adapters. Bands or single strips of tape do not obscure the connection site like wrapped tape does. Remember that a wrapped, obscured connection can still become disconnected, causing persistent bubbling in the water seal chamber as well as a pneumothorax.

Question: What are the most common causes of chest tube failure?
Answer: The most common causes of chest tube malfunction are too little suction, too much suction, and operator inexperience. Greater levels of suction may be warranted to enhance complete expansion of a stiff lung. Lower levels of suction may be warranted to avoid keeping a visceral pleural tear open. Low levels of suction or even a well-tolerated water seal can also allow the tear to heal before increasing suction to enhance complete lung reexpansion. In some cases both strategies are warranted. The important thing is for you to always have a management plan and a projected time table in mind when dealing with chest tubes and pathologic pleural processes.

Question: How do I troubleshoot my chest tubes?
Answer: Look for the problem, then solve it. Examine the chest drainage device for fluctuation or air leak in the water seal chamber, verify the amount of negative pressure being applied, remove kinks and loops from the chest tube, take down the dressing every 48 hours to examine the incision sites, verify skin

and suture integrity, and clean the area to avoid reactions to tape or adhesive.

Question: How do I remove a chest tube gracefully?

Answer: This is most easily done with an assistant. Both of you should wear sterile gloves. The chest tube site should be prepped with povidone-iodine. The securing sutures are carefully removed from the chest tube and severed. Ask the patient to hum or exhale forcefully as your assistant pulls the tube with one hand and closes the incision site with two fingers of the other hand. Then tie the resting suture to close the incision as it is gradually released by your assistant. Place the chest tube–drainage device ensemble into a biohazard bag. Clean the insertion site, wipe away all of the old tape, and place a clean, compressive dressing for 24 hours.

Question: How do I remove two chest tubes connected to a single thoracic drainage device by a Y connector?

Answer: Very carefully. Always clamp the first tube being removed so that air will not be aspirated into the pleural space through the other tube. If you are not removing both tubes that day, clamp the remaining tube so that the Y connector can be safely changed to a straight connector attaching the chest tube to the drainage device's rubber tubing. Don't forget to unclamp the tube before leaving the patient's bedside. In case of single chest tube removal, it does not matter whether the tube is clamped or unclamped. Nor does it matter whether suction is being applied.

Question: What if air enters the pleural space as I am removing the chest tube?

Answer: You probably noticed the gasping or sucking sound made as air was pulled through the chest wall incision into the patient's pleural space (ignore the "oh no" gasp of the operator). But you can fix this! Instead of tying the sutures tight immediately, the incision site should be pinched between two fingers. Rotate the patient so that the incision is facing uppermost, and ask the patient to perform a Valsalva maneuver. Gently release the incision site as the patient bears down. As air is expulsed from the pleural space you will hear a soft hissing sound. This maneuver can be repeated until all air has been evacuated.

✔ Procedural Guidelines: Large-Bore Chest Tube Insertion

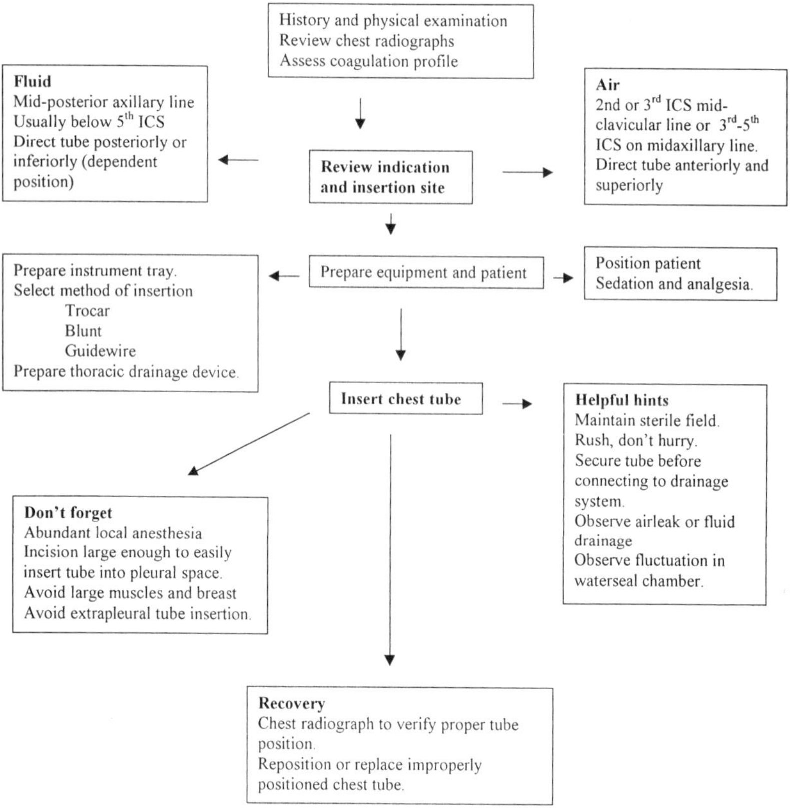

➧ Recommended Reading

Davis JW, Mackersie RC, Hoyt DB, Garcia J. Randomized study of algorithms for discontinuing tube thoracostomy drainage. J Am Coll Surg 1994;179:553–557.

Both suction and water seal algorithms had similar incidences of recurrent pneumothorax.

Gift AG, Bolgiano CS, Cunningham J. Sensations during chest tube removal. Heart Lung 1991;20:131–137.

Actually, the sensations experienced by patients are different from those described in standard nursing textbooks.

Mares DC, Mathur PN. Tube thoracostomy. J Bronchol 1997;4: 159–167.

A very detailed overview of chest tubes and insertion techniques.

Maurer JR, Friedman PJ, Wing VW. Thoracostomy tube in an interlobar fissure: radiologic recognition of a potential problem. AJR 1982;139:1155–1161.

The oblique position of a chest tube in the major fissure should not go unrecognized.

Miller SK, Sahn SA. Chest tubes: indications, technique, management, and complications. Chest 1987;91:258–264.

Contains a description of the three-bottle system and physiology of gas movement through tubing.

Munnell ER. Thoracic drainage. Ann Thorac Surg 1997;63:1497–1502.

A well-written, recent review by a thoracic surgeon.

14. BEDSIDE PLEURODESIS

✣ Definition

Pleurodesis, also known as pleural sclerosis, consists of permanent apposition of visceral and parietal pleural surfaces by chemical, mineral, or mechanical means. The goals of pleurodesis are (1) to prevent recurrence of pleural effusions; (2) to avoid subsequent thoracenteses or need for repeated chest tube insertions; (3) to provide long-lasting symptomatic relief; (4) to avoid morbidity related to recurrent pleural effusions or pneumothorax (trapped lung, atelectasis, pneumonia, respiratory insufficiency, tension pneumothorax); and (5) to improve quality of life and activity of daily living.

❍ Indications

- Rapidly recurrent malignant or benign pleural effusions despite large volume thoracentesis, unresponsive to systemic therapy. Ideal candidates have satisfactory performance levels (Karnofsky scores 40 or above), have an estimated survival greater than 3 months, and have demonstrated symptomatic improvement after thoracentesis with recurrence of symptoms after fluid reaccumulation.
- Recurrent spontaneous or secondary pneumothoraces, or first-time pneumothorax in patients at high risk for recurrence or in whom recurrent pneumothorax could result in substantial morbidity or mortality.

● Contraindications

- Patients with an expected survival of less than 3 months.
- Patients without symptoms attributable to the pleural effusion.
- Selected patients who may still benefit from systemic therapy (breast cancer, for example).
- Patients who refuse hospitalization or chest discomfort from tube thoracostomy.
- Patients with incomplete lung reexpansion following complete removal of pleural fluid (trapped lung).

❖ Equipment and Pleurodesis Agents

Pleurodesis is performed at the bedside via a tube thoracostomy after instillation of sclerosing agents (cytotoxic agents, tetracycline derivatives, or talc slurry) through an indwelling chest tube at the bedside.

Frequently used cytotoxic agents include **bleomycin** (40 to 80 units) and **mitoxantrone** (30 mg). The drug is usually combined with 30 to 100 cm^3 of normal saline solution. Success rates of 40% to 70% have been reported.

Frequently used tetracycline derivatives include **minocycline** (300 mg) and **doxycycline** (500 to 1,000 mg). The drug is usually combined with 30 to 100 cm^3 of normal saline solution and 20 mL of 2% lidocaine (Xylocaine). Success rates of 40% to 80% have been reported.

Talc is increasingly recognized as a most effective agent for pleurodesis, particularly for patients with recurrent malignant pleural effusions. Asbestos-free, United States Pharmacopeia (USP)–approved talc powder can be either purchased in bulk and sterilized in the hospital pharmacy, or prepackaged in sterile containers. It also comes in a single-use, disposable sterile aerosol container. For thoracoscopic insufflation, 2 to 4 g is usually used. Talc powder is insufflated through a pleural cannula using a pneumatic atomizer or aerosol container so that all pleural surfaces are covered. For slurry (talc is diluted in 100 milliliters of sterile normal saline solution), 5 to 10 g is used. Success rates greater than 90% are reported.

Bedside Pleurodesis Techniques

Before

If not previously inserted, a chest tube should be placed so that all of the pleural fluid can be evacuated. Ideally, the tube lies in a posterior and inferior position. The chest radiograph is reviewed to verify that the lung has fully expanded. Patients are warned that they may experience some chest discomfort as the chest tube is disconnected and the sclerosing agent is instilled. Premedication with meperidine (Demerol) 50 to 75 mg and/or hydroxyzine (Vistaril) 25 to 50 mg, or an anxiolytic agent, is often helpful. The patient is comfortably positioned in the partial lateral decubitus position, chest tube side up, and a towel is placed between the patient and the bed. **Material necessary for pleurodesis** is placed on a side table. This includes sterile gloves, a sterile drape, the sclerosing agent, 20 mL of 2% lidocaine, a sterile bottle of normal saline solution, a 60-cm^3 bulb syringe, a sterile bowl, sterile gauze, povidone-iodine solution, and two large chest tube clamps.

During

The chest tube is clamped with the two clamps and is disconnected from the adapter and suction tubing of the drainage device.

The clamps are briefly released, allowing the lung to collapse slightly within the pleural space. The lidocaine is instilled through the chest tube and the clamps are again placed. Using sterile technique, the sclerosing agent is mixed with saline solution in the sterile bowl and aspirated into the 60-cm^3 bulb syringe. If using talc, it is helpful to first pour the talc powder into the sterile saline bottle and to "shake it up" before pouring it into the bowl (Fig. 14-1). This keeps the talc from clumping. The syringe is attached to the chest tube, and the solution is instilled through the chest tube after both clamps have been removed. Once all of the solution is instilled, the patient is allowed to take a few breaths, with the chest tube unclamped, so that all of the solution is pulled into the pleural space. The tube is again clamped and connected to the suction device using the adapter. Connections are sealed using a banding gun. If possible, the patient can be gently rotated in bed (supine, and both partial lateral decubitus positions) during the next 2 hours, after which the clamps are removed, and the patient is once again connected to suction.

After

Two hours after pleurodesis, all clamps are removed and suction is reapplied. Additional analgesia is administered if necessary. A portable anteroposterior chest radiograph is obtained to assure lung reexpansion. Vital signs are monitored. The chest tube may

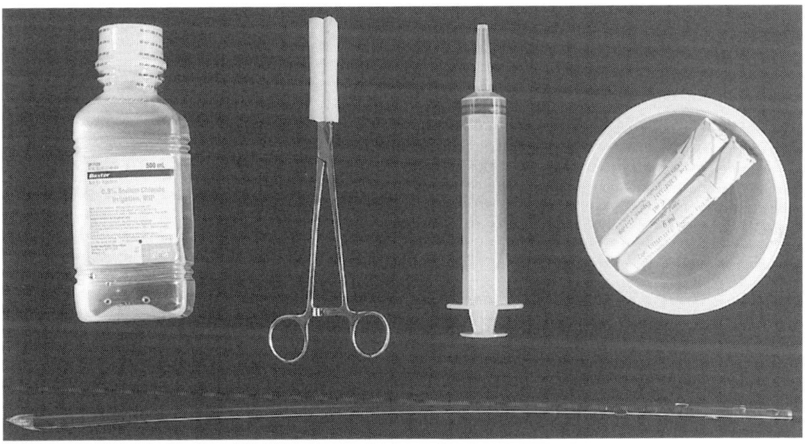

FIG. 14-1. Bedside talc slurry pleurodesis requires *(top, left to right)* sterile saline solution, a chest tube clamp, a sterile 60-cm^3 catheter tip syringe, a sterile bowl, sterile talc powder, and, preferably, *(below)* a large-bore chest tube.

be removed when daily pleural drainage decreases to less than 100 cm^3 or fluctuation is no longer visible in the water seal chamber, suggesting that the tube is no longer functional. Milking the chest tube twice a day may help to avoid fibrin deposition and tube clogging.

The ideal pleurodesis note should contain (1) a brief description of the procedure, including indication and techniques used; (2) the dose and type of sclerosing agent used; (3) the dose and type of analgesics or sedatives administered; and (4) a description of vital signs and patient tolerance of the procedure.

▼ Complications

- Pain is uncommon and can usually be alleviated by prophylactic administration of analgesics and sedatives. Pain occurs at the time of pleurodesis and usually does not linger for hours afterward.
- Tachycardia, tachypnea, and pneumonitis or respiratory failure have been described, particularly after talc slurry administration. No causal relationship has been demonstrated, and patients may have actually had reexpansion pulmonary edema. Any complications should be treated aggressively since they are usually reversible.
- Fever occurs in more than 30% of patients undergoing talc pleurodesis. This is probably related to temporary pleuritis, lasts for less than 48 hours, and is rarely associated with clinical symptoms. Blood cultures are usually unnecessary, but if fever persists, pleural fluid and blood cultures should be obtained and antibiotics administered.
- Incomplete lung expansion and partially trapped lung can result when pleurodesis is partially successful and the lung does not fully expand to fill the pleural cavity. In these cases, patients may describe shortness of breath for days, weeks, or months after the procedure. Incomplete lung reexpansion can be avoided by assuring proper chest tube position, full reexpansion immediately after pleurodesis, and by gradually increasing negative suction, even to levels greater than 20 cm H_2O as needed.

☆ Clinical Pearls

- Premedication with meperidine (50 to 100 mg IM) and hydroxyzine (25 to 50 mg IM) at least 30 minutes before pleurodesis can help alleviate procedure-associated pain.
- Addition of 20 mL of 2% to 4% lidocaine injected through the chest tube prior to administration of the sclerosing agent may also help alleviate procedure-related pain.

- Although pleurodesis can be performed through small-bore chest tubes, these clog easily so that larger bore tubes are preferred, particularly if talc is used.
- Pleurodesis is likely to fail if the chest tube is poorly positioned or is within the fissure. These chest tubes should probably be repositioned to enhance complete lung expansion before pleurodesis is attempted.

Heard on the Wards

Question: Does talc cause cancer?
Answer: No, unless it is contaminated with asbestos. To our knowledge, all currently marketed USP-approved talc powder is asbestos-free.

Question: Do results of pleurodesis depend on the agent used?
Answer: Yes. Review of the results of several recent studies pertaining to malignant pleural effusions demonstrate that talc, bleomycin, and doxycycline, for example, have success rates of greater than 90% (Viallat et al.), 79% (Zimmer et al.) and 65% (Heffner et al.), respectively. However, variations in study designs, doses used, methods of administration, and outcome measures render comparative analyses of the long-term efficacy of these agents difficult.

Question: Why is tetracycline no longer used?
Answer: Because of impurities. The intravenous solution no longer met Food and Drug Administration regulations, so Lederle Pharmaceuticals withdrew it from the market.

Question: What is talc slurry?
Answer: Talc slurry is a mixture of talc powder and sterile saline solution that is easily drawn into a syringe for instillation through a chest tube or directly into the pleural space for pleurodesis. "Shaken, not stirred" is the secret to a good slurry in which talc does not clump up in a mixing bowl or in the syringe. Effectiveness in preventing recurrent malignant pleural effusions is probably greater than 90% at 3 months.

Question: How do I treat someone with a large air leak who does not tolerate water seal after chemical or talc slurry pleurodesis?
Answer: If the patient cannot tolerate a clamped chest tube or water seal (because of a large air leak, for example), the clamps

are removed after you have raised the chest tubing and draped it over an IV pole. In this manner, suction can be applied without removing the sclerosing agent from the pleural space.

Question: Should patients be rotated after bedside pleurodesis?

Answer: Frankly, no one knows for sure. Do what you think is most logical until several well-designed studies have answered the question. Normally, one could assume that the pleurodesis agent will be equally distributed over all pleural surfaces as the lung expands and adheres uniformly to the parietal pleura.

Question: Is pleurodesis painful? If so, how do I avoid causing pain?

Answer: Pleurodesis can be painful if underlying parietal pleura is normal, as is usually the case in patients with pneu-

✔ Procedural Guidelines: Bedside Pleurodesis

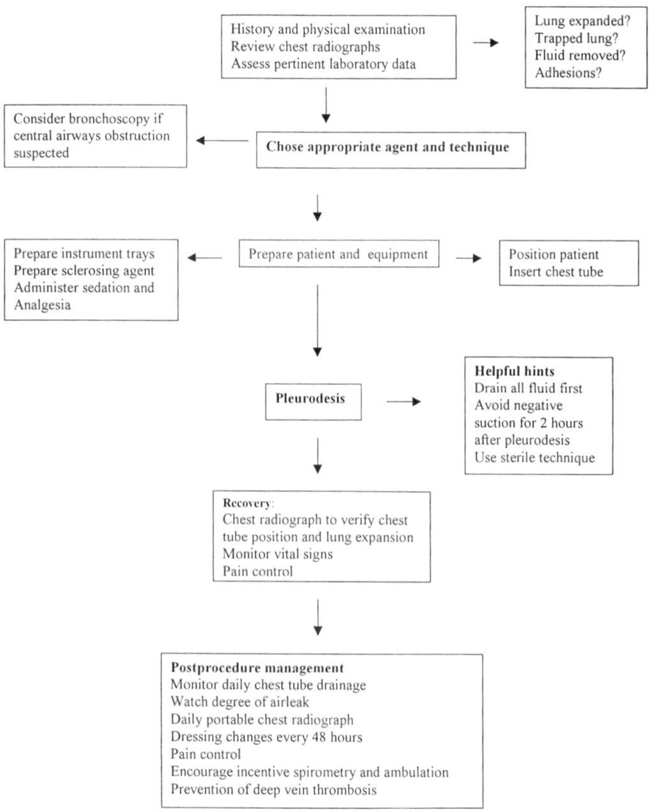

mothorax. Talc seems to cause far less pain than the tetracycline derivatives. Fifteen milliliters of 2% lidocaine can be combined with the pleurodesis agent to lessen discomfort, but it may not be as effective as parenteral narcotics such as meperidine 25 to 100 mg IM, sedatives such as hydroxyzine 25 to 50 mg IM, or anxiolytics such as midazolam 1 to 5 mg IV. Vital signs should be carefully monitored during and for at least 4 hours after pleurodesis if any of these drugs are used.

Recommended Reading

Colt HG. Thoracoscopic management of malignant pleural effusions. Clin Chest Med 1995;16:505–518.

Indications, techniques, and results are presented.

Hartman DL, Gaither JM, Kesler KA, Mylet DM, Brown JW, Mathur PN. Comparison of insufflated talc under thoracoscopic guidance with standard tetracycline and bleomycin pleurodesis for control of malignant pleural effusions. J Cardiovasc Surg 1993;105:743–748.

Talc was more effective (95% success at 90 days) than the other two sclerosing agents.

Heffner JE, Standerfer RJ, Torstveit J, Unruh L. Clinical efficacy of doxycycline for pleurodesis. Chest 1994;105:1743–1747.

Long-term efficacy was only 65% for malignant effusions. Most patients need at least two administrations of the drug.

Sanchez-Armengol A, Rodriguez-Panadero F. Survival and talc pleurodesis in metastatic pleural carcinoma, revisited. Report of 125 cases. Chest 1993;104:1482–1485.

Potential survival and response to pleurodesis may be related to pleural fluid pH and extent of pleural carcinomatosis as noted on thoracoscopic examination.

Viallat JR, Rey F, Astoul P, Boutin C. Thoracoscopic talc poudrage pleurodesis for malignant effusions: a review of 360 cases. Chest 1996;110:1387–1393.

Experience using talc pleurodesis from a French team having one of the most extensive experiences with thoracoscopy in the world.

Walker-Rennard PB, Vaughan LM, Sahn SA. Chemical pleurodesis for malignant pleural effusions. Ann Intern Med 1994;120: 56–64.

A review of multiple agents.

Zimmer PW, Hill M, Casey K, Harvey E, Low DE. Prospective randomized trial of talc slurry vs. bleomycin in pleurodesis for symptomatic malignant pleural effusions. Chest 1997;112: 430–434.

Another study showing that talc is the agent of choice.

15. THORACOSCOPY

✤ Definition

Direct or videoscopic inspection of the pleural space and lung using a rigid telescope inserted through small incisions made along the lateral chest wall, and through which parietal or visceral pleura can be sampled, fluid or air may be evacuated, and pleurodesis achieved. Procedures done under general anesthesia with selective double-lumen intubation, or procedures similar to those otherwise performed through an open thoracotomy, are often referred to as video-assisted thoracoscopic surgery (VATS).

❍ Indications

- Exudative or transudative pleural effusions of unclear etiology.
- Pneumothorax.
- Early empyema and complicated parapneumonic effusions.
- Hemothorax (although exploratory thoracotomy may be necessary).
- Pleural thickening of unclear etiology.
- Pleurodesis of recurrent effusions or pneumothorax.
- To obtain parietal pleura or lung biopsies for diagnosis of pleuropulmonary disorders including, but not limited to, primary or metastatic pleural carcinomatosis, malignant mesothelioma, tuberculosis or other granulomatous pleural disease, and infectious or interstitial lung disease of unclear etiology.

● Contraindications

- Inability to tolerate the lateral decubitus position.
- Unstable cardiovascular or hemodynamic status.
- Presence of severe, uncorrectable hypoxemia despite supplemental oxygenation.
- If general anesthesia and intubation are planned, thoracoscopy may not be warranted if patients cannot tolerate single-lung ventilation. This may be the case in critically ill, hypoxemic patients who are already on mechanical ventilation, or in patients with stiff, noncompliant lungs from advanced interstitial or infectious lung disease.
- Simple thoracoscopy is contraindicated if the pleural space cannot be easily accessed. This may be the case in patients with advanced empyema, pleural thickening of unknown

etiology, or suspected mesothelioma where the visceral and parietal pleural surfaces are fused.

❖ Equipment

Thoracoscopy can actually be performed with a very limited number of instruments. These include a small instrument tray containing a scalpel, scissors, hemostats, towel clamps, sutures, a needle driver, and forceps; at least one rigid Hopkins zero degree **telescope;** a fiberoptic light cable; 10-mm, 7-mm, and 5-mm pleural trocars and cannulas; a sponge forceps to clean the cannulas; a 5-mm electrocautery cupped biopsy forceps; an electrocautery cable; an electrosurgical unit; and a pneumatic atomizer for thoracoscopic talc insufflation (also known as talc poudrage) (Fig. 15-1). These instruments are easily placed on a sterile field set up on a large Mayo stand. A rubber tracheal or nasogastric suction canal can be used for aspirating pleural fluid, and a 28- to 32-Fr straight silicone chest tube should be inserted to evacuate residual air or fluid from the pleural space

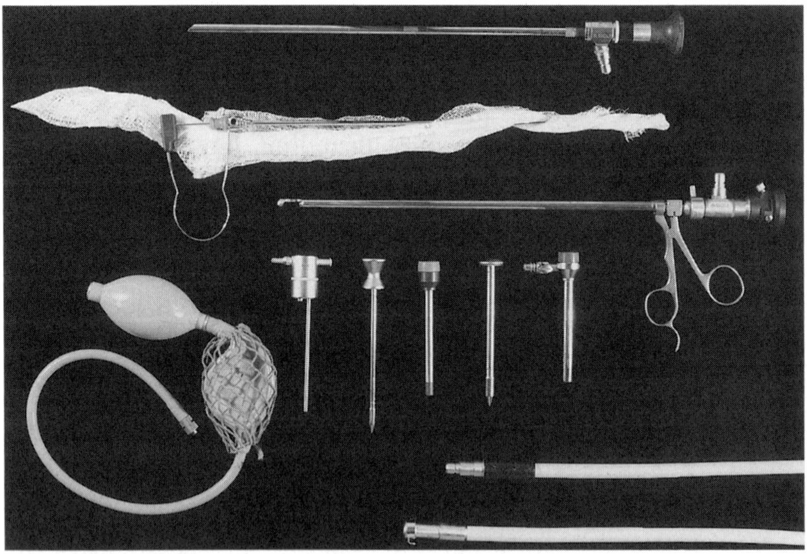

FIG. 15-1. Examples of basic instrumentation (Richard Wolf Inc.) used for diagnostic thoracoscopy or pleurodesis of a recurrent pleural effusion include a 7-mm telescope, sponge forceps used to clean inside of cannulas, 5-mm optical biopsy forceps, pleural trocars and cannulas, pneumatic atomizer for talc insufflation, and light cable *(top to bottom).*

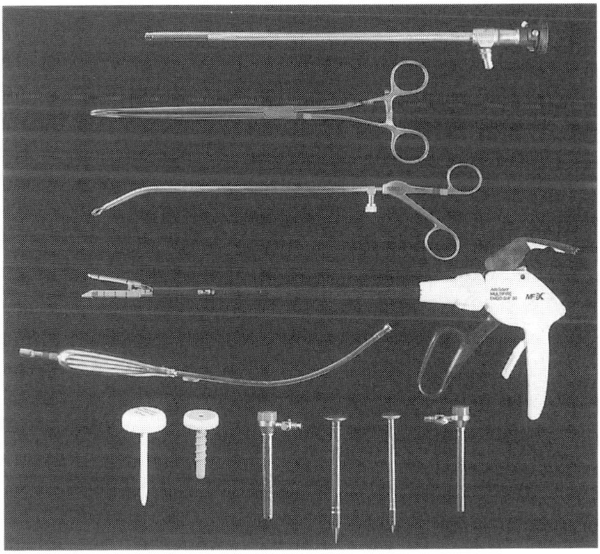

FIG. 15-2. Examples of basic instrumentation used for thoracoscopic lung biopsy include 10-mm telescope, ring forceps (Pilling-Rusch), atraumatic 7-mm grasping forceps (Richard Wolf Inc.), endoscopic stapling device (United States Surgical Corporation Autosuture), Yankaur suction device, and several disposable or reusable trocars and cannulas *(top to bottom).*

and reexpand the lung at the end of the procedure. Ideally, a high-powered xenon or cold light source, a **video camera** that fits easily onto the eyepiece of the rigid telescope, a video recorder, a video display screen, and a video cart are available. For certain procedures, grasping forceps and instruments adapted from open thoracic surgical interventions are also desirable (Fig. 15-2). An external electrosurgery device (Bovie unit) should be available in case electrocauterization of adhesions or biopsy sites is warranted. If thoracoscopy through a single access site is envisioned, a 7-mm optical biopsy forceps (with its 4-mm 5-degree rigid telescope) or a 10-mm bayonet thoracoscope (with its 5-mm accessory instrument channel and 5-mm rigid telescope) is warranted.

◆ Techniques

Regardless of the technique employed, the following **seven simple rules** govern safe thoracoscopy: (1) the first incision should provide intrapleural access; (2) trocars should not be blindly inserted into the pleural space. Rather, it is best to make a wider incision, and to gently insert an index finger into the pleural space to push the adherent lung away from the chest wall and induce a partial, controlled, open pneumothorax; (3) additional trocars and cannulas should be inserted under videothoracoscopic guidance; (4) unknown or unrecognized intrapleural structures should never be biopsied; (5) sufficient analgesia and sedation should be provided to assure a pain-free procedure; (6) a chest tube is always inserted at the end of the procedure and connected to a thoracic drainage device to assure complete lung reexpansion and evacuation of the pneumothorax; (7) circulating personnel should be available to help manipulate instruments, maintain the patient's safety and comfort, and assist as needed, particularly in case of equipment malfunction.

Before

Once in the lateral decubitus position, involved side facing upward, an axillary roll ("bolster") is placed beneath the patient to increase the size of the intercostal spaces. The bolster should not be placed too high in the axilla so as to avoid injuring the brachial plexus or compromising blood circulation. The patient is secured in the lateral decubitus position using rolled towels wrapped with sticky material, with a bead bag, pillows, or lateral supports placed on either side of the patient (Fig. 15-3). A pillow

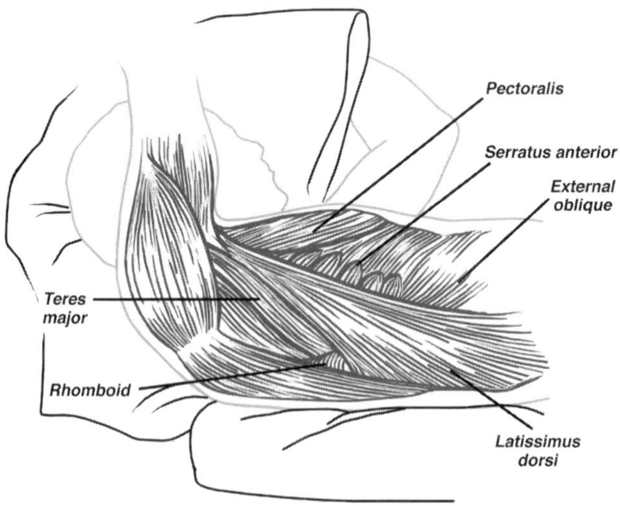

FIG. 15-3. Patient in left lateral decubitus position. Thoracoscopy can be performed via 1-cm incisions through the serratus anterior (lateral ports) and pectoralis major (anterior ports) muscles.

is placed between the legs of the patient, and care is taken to avoid excess pressure on bony structures, fragile skin, or the brachial plexus. Intercostal incision sites are marked with a sterile pen. The lateral chest is prepped and draped in the usual sterile fashion.

The operator usually stands in front of the patient because the majority of parietal pleura pathology is found along the posterior costal pleura. The assistant stands behind the patient. The procedure nurse has set up the necessary instruments on a Mayo stand over the patient, with additional instruments available on an adjacent procedure table. A circulating nurse is responsible for the organization of the procedure room, for setting up the video equipment, and for providing additional instruments that may be needed. The anesthesiologist standing behind the sterile drapes at the head of the patient is responsible for the patient's anesthesia, ventilation, oxygenation, and analgesia.

During

Thoracoscopy can be performed under **local anesthesia supplemented by intravenous administration** of narcotics and neuroleptics. In this case, procedures should be limited to inspection of the pleura and lung, evacuation of pleural effusions, and performance of parietal pleural biopsies or pleurodesis. Spontaneous, nonassisted ventilation is usually unimpaired, although the awake patient may not be fully cooperative. Breathing, which is often labored prior to removal of pleural fluid, actually improves during the procedure. The open, controlled pneumothorax is almost always well tolerated, and partial lung collapse facilitates satisfactory visualization of surrounding pleural and chest wall structures. Using this technique, duration of procedures should be under 30 minutes.

Abundant **local anesthesia** should be administered to the incision sites, which should be kept small. The first incision should be made along the 5th or 6th intercostal space on the midaxillary line. After insertion of the trocar and cannula, pleural fluid is removed and inspection with a rigid telescope is performed (Fig. 15-4). If necessary, a second **incision** is made more inferiorly and either anteriorly or posteriorly for insertion of another trocar and cannula under videothoracoscopic guidance. If the pleural territory to be biopsied is posterior, the access site should be anterior; if, on the other hand, the pleural territory for biopsy is anterior, the access site should be posterior and directly across from the target area. Additional sedation or analgesia is necessary at the time of pleural biopsy. Parietal **pleural**

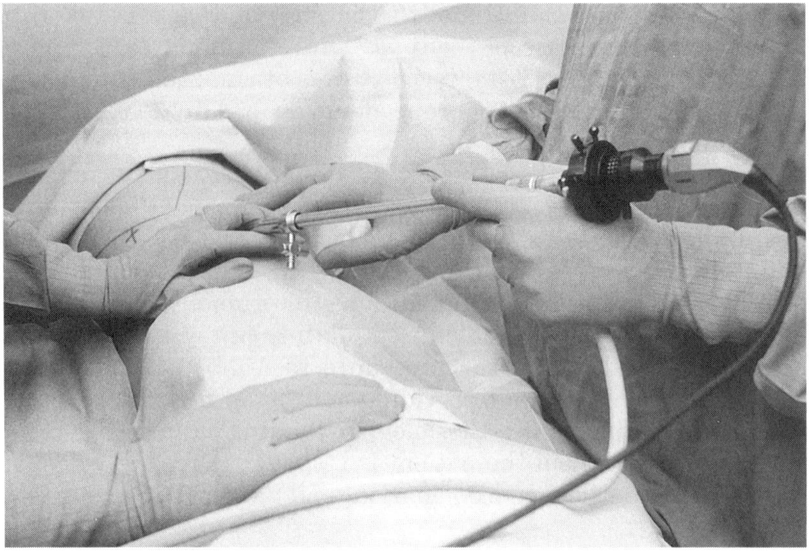

FIG. 15-4. Camera attached to telescope via standard C mount. Thoracoscopy is performed through 7th intercostal space midaxillary line. Note additional point of entry drawn on lateroposterior chest wall.

biopsies are readily taken using 5-mm electrocautery forceps (Fig. 15-5). Specimens are obtained from parietal pleura immediately overlying the indurated, bony surface of a rib to avoid biopsying the intercostal neurovascular bundle. **Specimens** should not be obtained from the apex of the hemithorax (too many vascular structures), the anterior parietal pleura, particularly in proximity to the internal mammary artery, or if thickened parietal pleura masks underlying neurovascular structures. Manipulation of the lung should be avoided because it may cause cough or chest discomfort, or result in visceral pleural tears. Because **pleurodesis** by thoracoscopic talc insufflation is occasionally painful, closing sutures should be placed through incision sites and the mandatory chest tube prepared before insufflating the talc onto the pleural surfaces.

Thoracoscopy is also performed under **general anesthesia after single or double-lumen intubation**.This technique is warranted (1) in patients in whom it is feared that excessive sedation or neuroleptic anesthesia will be poorly tolerated or result in respiratory insufficiency; (2) if manipulation of the lung is expected; or (3) if a multiloculated pleural space is expected and

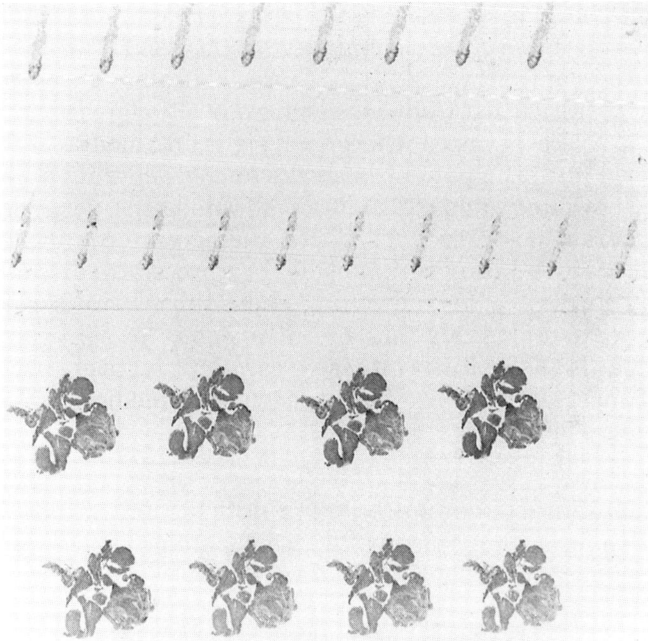

FIG. 15-5. Final processing and hematoxylin-eosin staining of parietal pleural shows size differences of specimens obtained by closed-needle biopsy *(top)* and thoracoscopic forceps biopsy *(bottom)*.

adhesions will need to be severed using combinations of sharp and blunt dissection. Although the expense of these procedures is higher (costs of operating room suite and anesthesia), multiple diagnostic and therapeutic procedures are possible, making this an excellent alternative for many patients and physicians. In case of intubation, the position of the endotracheal tube should always be verified by flexible fiberoptic bronchoscopy before and after the patient has been placed in the full lateral decubitus position.

The first **access** site is usually made in the 5th to 7th intercostal space on the midaxillary line. The pleural space is inspected, and additional trocars and cannulas inserted under videothoracoscopic guidance. Ideally, two or three access sites are made in triangular fashion (e.g., the 7th, 4th, and 5th intercostal spaces on the mid-, anterior, and posterior axillary lines). Sufficient space between these sites should allow the operator to avoid dueling instruments. At the end of the procedure, incision sites are closed in layers using absorbable sutures, and the skin is closed using an absorbable subcuticular running stitch or by separate mattress sutures using 2.0 or 3.0 nylon. The chest tube is secured and attached to a thoracic drainage device. The patient is turned back onto the supine position, extubated, and moved to a recovery area where vital signs and mental status are monitored until the patient is awake and stable from a hemodynamic, ventilatory, and oxygenation standpoint. A portable anterior-posterior postprocedure chest radiograph confirms chest tube position and lung reexpansion. Postprocedure discomfort is usually caused by the indwelling chest tube. Pain is well controlled with oral analgesics or intravenous patient-controlled analgesia. Transfer to an intensive care unit is rarely necessary, so that most patients are hospitalized on a medical or surgical ward (Fig. 15-6).

After

The ideal thoracoscopy procedure note should include (1) the indication for the procedure; (2) a brief summary of the patient's

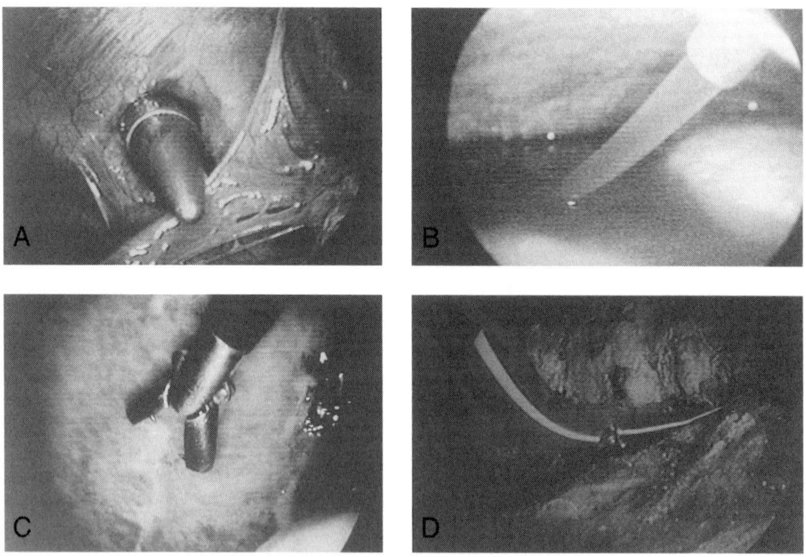

FIG. 15-6. Videothoracoscopic photographs showing **(A)** pleural trocar and cannula inserted adjacent to an adhesion; **(B)** aspiration of pleural fluid using a flexible, atraumatic catheter (note collapsed lung bathing in pleural fluid); **(C)** parietal pleural biopsy using 5-mm toothed forceps in a patient with sarcoidosis; and **(D)** large-bore chest tube in place after talc pleurodesis. Note sentinel hole cut on radiopaque line.

pleuropulmonary disease history with pertinent clinical and laboratory findings (pleural fluid analysis, results of radiographic imaging, pertinent other diagnoses, clinical course leading to thoracoscopy); (3) the operator and assistant's names; (4) the mode of anesthesia or sedation used; (5) location (operating room or procedure suite); (6) the patient's position and number of points of entry; (7) the location of trocar insertion sites; (8) a detailed description of the intervention and diagnostic or therapeutic procedures performed; (9) the amount of pleural fluid and source of biopsy specimens removed; (10) a description of any adverse events and their impact on patient outcome; (11) a description of the patient's clinical status after the procedure; and (12) results of the postprocedure chest radiograph.

▼ Complications

- Procedure-related mortality is rare if satisfactory precautions are taken. These include careful monitoring of vital signs such as heart rate, blood pressure, cardiac rhythm, and oxygen saturation; avoiding excessive sedation or respiratory insufficiency in the nonintubated patient; and paying careful attention to both normal and abnormal anatomic structures before grasping, mobilizing, or biopsying anything in the thorax.
- Laceration of intercostal vessels can be avoided by keeping skin incisions superficial and small, carefully dilating incision sites before introducing pleural trocars and cannulas, not inserting sharp-edged trocars (several disposable laparoscopic trocars are sharp-edged), and always biopsying parietal pleura overlying a rib rather than overlying an intercostal space.
- Laceration of lung parenchyma can be avoided by not inserting trocars briskly or blindly through incision sites, dilating the first point of entry sufficiently to allow introduction of an index finger to manually palpate the lung and parietal pleural adjacent to the incision site, and bluntly severing adhesions before pushing the lung gently away from the chest wall. Additional trocars and cannulas should be inserted under videothoracoscopic guidance. In addition, the lung should only be grasped with atraumatic forceps and without applying excess traction or rotation to the parenchyma.
- Intrathoracic vascular injury is avoided by never biopsying an area without being absolutely certain of anatomic relationships, dissecting adhesions only when necessary,

paying careful attention to the anterior chest wall (territory of the internal mammary artery) and apex (territory of the carotid and subclavian vessels), and by avoiding undue manipulation of the lung deep in the fissures or in areas surrounding mediastinal and hilar vessels.

- Rib fractures are caused by undue pressure during patient positioning or trocar insertion in frail patients with metastatic bone disease.
- Cervical spine fractures are caused by undue rotation during patient positioning, particularly in patients with metastatic bone involvement or unstable cervical spines.
- Cutaneous pressure sores or brachial plexus injuries are caused by improper positioning and inadequate use of pads and cushions on pressure-sensitive areas.
- Empyema or subcutaneous abscesses are avoided by using sterile technique and avoiding contamination of trocar insertion sites with contaminated material.
- Postprocedure chest discomfort is avoided by using generous local anesthesia at incision and chest tube insertion sites. Adequate analgesia after thoracoscopy is maintained by using appropriate intravenous and oral narcotics. Remember these drugs can cause respiratory depression, drowsiness, constipation, and urinary dysfunction.
- Tumor seeding of the operative site and trocar insertion sites, particularly in patients with malignant mesothelioma, can usually be avoided by delivering external beam irradiation (21 Gy delivered to 3-cm insertion depths over 3 days) to the incision sites 10 to 14 days after thoracoscopy.
- Incomplete lung expansion after thoracoscopy can usually be avoided by careful positioning of one or two chest tubes as needed under videothoracoscopic guidance, proper management of thoracic drainage devices, adequate use of analgesics to avoid chest splinting during inspiration and expiration, and supervised use of incentive spirometry. Early ambulation should be encouraged.

☆ Clinical Pearls

- A careful history and physical should always be performed to identify disease states that may affect management. These include, but are not limited, to (1) unstable cervical spine (from arthritis or metastatic bone disease) that could make lateral decubitus positioning dangerous; (2) underlying heart disease, including arrhythmias; (3) bladder, prostate, or renal dysfunction; (4) coagulopathy; (6) occult neoplasm, such as colon, breast, stomach, or malignant melanoma; (7) thyroid disease; (8) anxiety or depression; (9) obstructive pulmonary disease; and (10) constipation.

- Points of entry can be drawn on the lateral chest before placing sterile drapes. The strategy of trocar placement depends on the procedure being performed.
- Although the first point of entry should be large enough to allow introduction of an index finger into the pleural cavity, additional incision sites should be kept as small as possible, and trocars inserted under videothoracoscopic visualization.
- If applying suction during the procedure, the lung will expand unless enough air can enter the pleural cavity through another incision or cannula.
- Postprocedure incentive spirometry enhances complete lung expansion, secretion clearance, and improves atelectasis.

Heard on the Wards

Question: When is open lung biopsy preferable to thoracoscopic lung biopsy?

Answer: Open lung biopsy is preferable to thoracoscopic lung biopsy in patients who would not tolerate single lung ventilation well enough to allow sufficient lung collapse and manipulation of an endoscopic stapling device. This may be the case in patients with increasing hypoxemia and stiff, noncompliant lungs who have been on mechanical ventilation. Thoracotomy may also be preferred if the patient has a bleeding disorder.

Question: What are the most feared complications of thoracoscopy and how are they avoided?

Answer: Proper training, careful technique, and experience are the keys to a safe procedure. Complications may be procedure-related (puncture of the lung by blind insertion of a pleural trocar, inadvertent biopsy of an intercostal vessel), anesthesia-related (hypoxemia from inadequate intraoperative ventilation, prolonged atelectasis, or inappropriate use of drugs that inhibit the autoregulatory hypoxic pulmonary vasoconstriction during single-lung ventilation), or instrument-related (lung laceration from a defective endoscopic stapling device).

Question: What should I watch for while rounding on patients who have just had a thoracoscopy?

Answer: The attending! Always write a note, review the chest radiograph, and diligently monitor fluid drainage or presence of

✔ Procedural Guidelines: Thoracoscopy

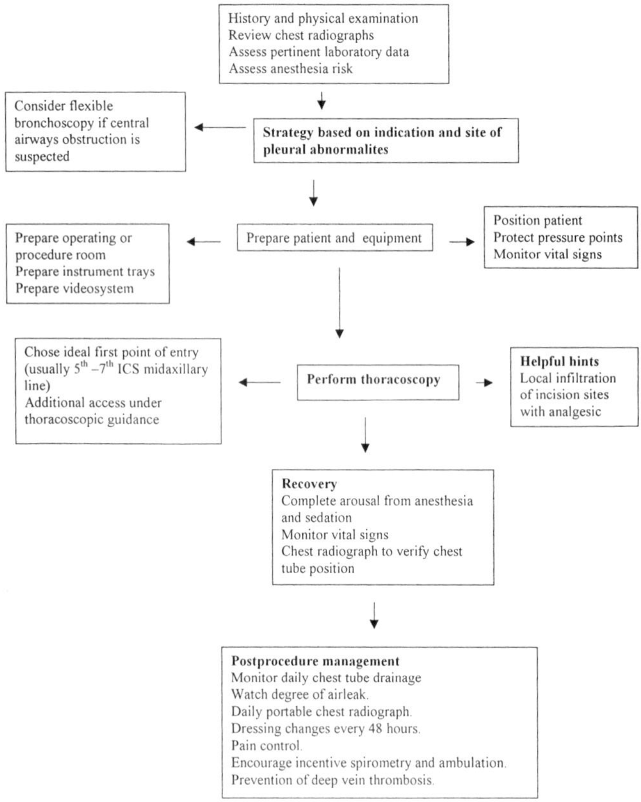

air leak in the chest drainage device. Chart vital signs, especially temperature and fluid status. Encourage early ambulation and incentive spirometry to avoid prolonged atelectasis. Treat pain aggressively. Pay attention to details that may impact on the patient's comfort. Communicate with each patient's family members and loved ones. Be a good listener. Most of all, do your best to be cheerful, positive, and realistically optimistic, especially if your patient has a malignancy or other life-threatening illness.

➧ Recommended Reading

Colt HG. Thoracoscopy: a prospective study of safety and outcome. Chest 1995;108:324–329.

Thoracoscopy was diagnostic in 93% of cases, and talc pleurodesis was effective in 91% of cases. Safety was addressed prospectively using a list of potential complications.

Davidson J, Colt HG. Thoracoscopy: nursing implications for optimal patient outcomes. Dimens Crit Care Nursing 1997;19: 20–28.

A review of what to watch out for during nursing care of patients after thoracoscopy.

Mathur PN, Loddenkemper R. Medical thoracoscopy: role in pleural and lung diseases. Clin Chest Med 1995;16:487–496.

A thorough review.

Menzies R, Charbonneau M. Thoracoscopy for the diagnosis of pleural disease. Ann Intern Med 1991;114:271–276.

Under local anesthesia, thoracoscopy was safe and effective. The negative predictive value for malignancy was 93%.

Thomas PA. A thoracoscopic peek: what did Jacobaeus see? Ann Thorac Surg 1994;57:770–771.

Hans Christian Jacobaeus, a Swedish physician, invented thoracoscopy more than 80 years ago.

Viallat JR, Rey F, Astoul P, Boutin C. Thoracoscopic talc poudrage pleurodesis for malignant effusions: a review of 360 cases. Chest 1996;110:1387–1393.

Experience using talc pleurodesis from a French team having one of the most extensive experiences with thoracoscopy in the world.

Weissberg D. Talc pleurodesis: experience with 360 patients. J Thorac Cardiovasc Surg 1993;106:689–695.

Excellent results noted in 90% of cases, including benign recurrent effusions and chylothorax.

APPENDIX

APPENDIX: **INSTRUMENT MANUFACTURERS**

Arrow International Inc. (Reading, PA)

Bauer Medical Inc. (Clearwater, FL)

Cook Inc. (Bloomington, IN)

Deknatel-Snowdon-Pencer (Fall River, MA)

Manan Medical Products (Northbrook, IL)

Medi-tech Boston Scientific Corporation (Watertown, MA)

Mill-Rose Laboratories, Inc. (Mentor, OH)

Pilling-Rusch (Ft. Washington, PA)

Richard Wolf Inc. (Vernon Hills, IL)

Sherwood, Davis, and Geck (St. Louis, MO)

Sherwood Medical (St. Louis, MO)

United States Surgical Corporation (Norwalk, CT)

Wilson-Cook Medical Inc. (Bloomington, IN)

SUBJECT INDEX

SUBJECT INDEX

Note: Figures and tables are represented by f and t respectively; page numbers in *italics* represent topics discussed in the question and answer section at the end of each chapter.

A

Abrams needle, for pleural biopsy, 106, 108, 108f
Acetaminophen, 68–69
  adverse effects, 69
Acoustic coupling, ultrasonographic, 37, 37f
Addiction, to opioids, 72–73, 74
Adhesions
  closed-tube thoracostomy and, *135*
  pleural ultrasonographic findings, *43*
Air
  in pleural radiology, 25, 25f, 32. *See also* Pneumothorax
  into pleural space, in closed-tube thoracostomy
    during insertion, *149*
    during removal, *151*
Air-fluid level, in pleural space, 29–30, 30f
Air hunger, in pleural disease, 13
Air leaks
  closed-tube thoracostomy and, 134–135
  treatment options, *159–160*
  in water seal chamber, 50
Alfentanyl, 72
Amitriptyline, 74
Amylase, pleural fluid, 80
Analgesia
  gate control theory, 67–68
  patient-controlled, *76*
Analgesics, 67–73
  adverse effects, 68. *See also individual agents*
  agents used as, 68–73
  contraindications, 68
  indications, 68
  principles of use, 67–68
  tapering use, 74
  tolerance to, 68
Anaphylactic shock, local anesthetics causing, 64
Anatomic landmarks
  for physical examination of chest
    during inspection, 14–16, 14f–16f
    during palpation, 16
  for thoracentesis, *9*
Angle of Louis, 3
Anterior intercostal arteries, 5
Antibiotics, prophylactic, prior to thoracoscopy, *75*
Antidepressants, 73–74
  adverse effects, 73
  agents used as, 74
  contraindications, 73
  indications, 73
  principles of use, 73
Antihistamines, 67
Antimicrobial ointments, topical. *See* Topical antimicrobial ointments
Antiseptics, defined, 53
Anxiolytics, 65–67
  adverse effects, 66
  agents used as, 66–67
  contraindications, 65–66
  indications, 65
  principles of use, 65
Argyle chest tubes, 139–140, 139f
Argyle-Turkel safety needle, for thoracocentesis, 93, 94f
  technique, 98
Argyle-Turkel safety pneumothorax catheter, 127, 128f
Arrow cavity drainage catheters, 128
Arrow pneumothorax set, 128, 129f
Arteries, intercostal, 5–6
Asbestos-related pleuropulmonary disease, 32
Aspirin, 69
Atelectasis, rounded, *33 34*
Ativan (lorazepam), 66
Auscultation
  in pleural effusions, 17
  in pneumothorax, 1
  technique, 16
Axillary lines

Axillary lines *(cont'd)*
described, *9–10*
lateral chest wall, 15–16, 16f

B
Bacitracin, topical application, 62
Banding gun, 146, 147f
Bedside pleurodesis. *See* Pleurodesis
Biopsy
closed-needle. *See* Closed-needle pleural biopsy
fine-needle. *See* Fine-needle aspiration biopsy
Blebs
versus bullae, *34–35*
in spontaneous pneumothorax, 83
Bleomycin, 156
B-mode ultrasonography, 37–38
Boutin needle, for thoracocentesis, 93, 94f
technique, 97–98
Bradycardia, opioids causing, 72
Breath sounds
descriptive terms for, *19*
in pleural effusions, 18
in pneumothorax, 18
Bronchopleural fistula, lung abscess versus, 30, *34*
Bronchoscopic lung biopsy, fine-needle aspiration biopsy versus, *124*
Bullae, blebs versus, *34–35*
Bupivacaine, 64

C
Calcifications, in pleural radiographic findings, 27
Capp's point, 19
Carbocaine hydrochloride (mepivacaine), 64
Cardiovascular toxicity, from local anesthetics, 63
Catamenial pneumothorax, *88*
Catheter-over-guidewire technique, 130, 131f, 132
Central airways obstruction, pleural effusions and, 26
Central nervous system toxicity, from local anesthetics, 63
Chest, anatomic landmarks
anterior, 14f
lateral chest wall, 16f
posterior, 15f
Chest pain, in pleural disease, 13
Chest radiographs
after chest drainage device set-up, 49
after closed-tube thoracostomy, 132f, 133, 133f, *149–150*
after thoracentesis, 98
views, 21
Chest tubes
for closed-tube thoracostomy
large-bore. *See under* Closed-tube thoracostomy
malfunction, *150*
in pleurodesis, 159
removal, *151*
small-bore. *See under* Closed-tube thoracostomy
troubleshooting for, *150–151*
drainage devices and. *See* Thoracic drainage devices
wounds from. *See* Wounds, chest tube
Chest wall
anatomy
anterolateral, 4, 4f
posterolateral, 4, 5f
physical examination, 13–20
in pleural radiology, 24
Chiba style needle, 116f–117f, 117
Chlorhexidine gluconate, 56
laundering and, 55
Chylothorax, 81, 84
Cidex (two percent glutaraldehyde), 57
Cleaning, defined, 54
Closed-needle pleural biopsy, 81, 105–113
complications, 111
contraindications, 105
defined, 105
documentation requirements, 110–111
equipment, 105–108, 106f–108f
indications, 105, *112–113*
procedural guidelines, 113
techniques, 108–111
Closed-tube thoracostomy
using large-bore chest tubes, 139–152
complications, 147–148
contraindications, 139
defined, 139
documentation requirements, 146–147
equipment, 139–140, 139f
indications, 139
insertion techniques, 140–142, 141f, 143f–147f, 144–147, 148–149
in loculated pleural effusion, 149
procedural guidelines, 152
size selection, 149
using small-bore chest tubes, 127–136
complications, 134
contraindications, 127
defined, 127

documentation requirements, 133–134
equipment, 127–128, 128f–130f, 130
indications, 127
insertion
techniques, 130, 131f–133f, 132–134
verification, *135*
procedural guidelines, 136
size selection, *135*
Cocaine, 64–65
Codeine, 71
Color Doppler ultrasonography, *42*
Computed tomography, 21–22
for fine-needle aspiration biopsy, 115, 120, 121f, *124*
Constipation, as opioid adverse effect, 72
treatment, *76*
Cook percutaneous chest tube sets, 128, 129f
Cope needle, for pleural biopsy, 105–106, 106f, 107f
safe use, *112*
Costodiaphragmatic recess
in pleural cavity anatomy, 7
in thoracic cage anatomy, 3
Costomediastinal recess, in thoracic cage anatomy, 3
Cough
in pleural disease, 13
thoracentesis and, 99, *100*
Crown biopsy needle, for fine-needle aspiration biopsy, 116–117, 116f–117f
CT. *See* Computed tomography
Cystic fibrosis, pleurodesis and, 83
Cytopathologist, prescence during biopsy, 123
Cytotoxic agents, 156

D

Dalmane (flurazepam), 66
Decontamination, defined, 53–54
Degerming, skin, 53–59. *See also* Skin degerming
Demerol (meperidine), 71
Diaphragm, in thoracic cage anatomy, 3
Diazepam, 66
Diclofenac, 69
Diflunisal, 69
Dilaudid (hydromorphone), 71
Disinfection, 53–59. *See also* Skin degerming
agents used for
labeling information, 58
washing off, 58
in closed-needle pleural biopsy, 109
complications, 58
defined, 53
in fine-needle aspiration biopsy, 120
handwashing and, 58
high-level, 53
agents used for, 57
techniques, 56
intermediate-level, 53
low-level, 53
in thoracentesis, 95
Documentation
chest drainage device surveillance, 21
closed-needle pleural biopsy, 110–111
closed-tube thoracostomy
using large-bore chest tubes, 146–147
using small-bore chest tubes, 133–134
fine-needle aspiration biopsy, 122
pleurodesis, 158
thoracentesis, 98–99
thoracic drainage devices, 49
thoracoscopy, 170–171
ultrasonography, 40
Dolobid (diflunisal), 69
Doxepin, 74
Doxycycline, 156
Drainage devices, thoracic, 45–52. *See also* Thoracic drainage devices
Dressings, for chest tube wounds, after closed-tube thoracostomy, 145–146, 147f
Dressler's syndrome, 84
"Dry tap," in thoracentesis, *101–102*
avoiding, *102*
Duragesic (fentanyl patch), 72
Dyspnea, in pleural disease, 13

E

Edema, reexpansion pulmonary, thoracentesis and, 99
Effusions
lamellar, 32
pleural. *See* Pleural effusions
Elastic recoil, lung, 8
Emerson pump, 45
Empiric therapy, for pleural effusion, 81
Empyema
defined, 82
radiographic findings, 30
treatment, 82
Endocarditis prophylaxis, *75*
EO gas sterilization, 57–58
Eosinophilia, in pleural fluid, 80
Epinephrine, contraindications, 63

Ethylene oxide sterilization, 57–58
Expiration, muscles of, 4, 5f
Expiration dates, on sterile packaging, *59*
External intercostal muscles, 5
Extrapleural disease, pleural abnormalities versus, 30–31, 31f
Extrapleural fat, in pleural radiographic findings, 28
Exudate
  defined, *10*
  in pleural effusion differential diagnosis, 79

F

Fasting, closed-needle pleural biopsy and, *112*
Fat, extrapleural, in pleural radiographic findings, 28
Feldene (piroxicam), 70
Fentanyl, 71–72
Fentanyl patch, 72
Fever, in pleural disease, 13
Fibrosis, pleural
  diffuse, 28
  radiographic findings, 27–28, 28f
Fibrothorax
  diagnosis, 83
  management, 83
Fine-needle aspiration biopsy, 115–125
  versus bronchoscopic lung biopsy, *124*
  complications, 122–123
  contraindications, 115
  defined, 115
  documentation requirements, 122
  equipment, 116–118, 116f–117f
  indications, 115, *124–125*
  procedural guidelines, 125
  techniques, 118–122, 121f, 124
Fissures, in pleural radiology, 23, 24f
  fluid in, 32
Fistula, bronchopleural, lung abscess versus, 30
Flash sterilization, 57
Fluid. *See* Pleural fluid
Flumazenil, 66–67
Fluoroscopy, for fine-needle aspiration biopsy, 115, 124, *124*
Flurazepam, 66
Formaldehyde, 57
Formalin (formaldehyde), 57
Franseen biopsy needle, for fine-needle aspiration biopsy, 116–117, 116f–117f
FRC. *See* Functional residual capacity
Free air, in pleural space, 29, 29f. *See also* Pneumothorax
Free-flowing pleural fluid
  in pleural radiographic findings, 26
  in pleural ultrasonographic findings, 39f, *42*
Frontal chest radiographs, 21
Functional residual capacity, lung, 7, 8

G

Gastric air bubble, in pleural radiology, 23
General anesthesia, for thoracoscopy, 168–169
Germicides, defined, 53
Glucose, pleural fluid, 80
Glutaraldehyde, two percent, 57
Gradient of pleural pressure, 8

H

Heimlich valve chest drainage device, 45, 47, 48f
Hemothorax
  causes, 82
  thoracentesis and, 99
  treatment, 82
Hexachlorophene, 55
Hibiclens (chlorhexidine gluconate), 56
  laundering and, 58
Hopkins zero degree telescope, 164
Hospitalization, after thoracoscopy, 170
Hyaline plaques, in pleural radiographic findings, 27–28
Hydrocodone, 71
Hydrogen peroxide, 55
Hydromorphone, 71
Hydropneumothorax, 29–30, 30f
Hydroxyzine, 67
  for pain alleviation in pleurodesis, 158
Hypersensitivity reactions, to local anesthetics, 64
Hypnotics, 65–67. *See also* Anxiolytics
Hypotension
  local anesthetics causing, 63
  opioids causing, 72

I

Ibuprofen, 69
Imipramine, 74
Indocin (indomethacin), 69
Indomethacin, 69
Infection, thoracentesis and, 99
Injection
  intramuscular. *See* Intramuscular administration
  intravenous. *See* Intravenous administration

local anesthetic, site for, 62–63
Inspection
anatomical landmarks for, 14–16, 14f–16f
in pleural effusions, 17
in pneumothorax, 18
Inspiration, muscles of, 4, 4f
Instrumentation
disinfection, 56
manufacturers for, 179
sterilization, 57–58. *See also* Sterilization
for thoracoscopy, 164–165, 164f–165f
Intercostal muscles, 5
Intercostal nerves, 6
Intercostal spaces
anatomy, 5–6
counting method, *19*
Intercostal vessels
arteries, 5–6
in thoracentesis, *10*
veins, 6
Internal intercostal muscles, 5
Intramuscular administration
morphine sulfate, 70–71
respiratory depression after, 74
Intravenous administration
morphine sulfate, 70–71
respiratory depression after, 74
Iodophores, 55
Isopropyl alcohol, 55

K
Kampmeier's foci, 8
Ketorolac, 70

L
Lamellar effusions, 32
Large-bore chest tubes, for closed-tube thoracostomy. *See under* Closed-tube thoracostomy
Lateral chest radiographs, 21
Laxatives, *76*
Left lung, 7
Lidocaine, 64
for pain alleviation in pleurodesis, 158
Light's criteria, in pleural effusion differential diagnosis, 79
Litten's sign, 19
Liver toxicity, acetaminophen causing, 69
Local anesthesia, for thoracoscopy, 167
Local anesthetics, 62–65
adverse effects, 63–64
agents used in, 64–65
contraindications, 62
dosage, 62
indications, 62
principles of use, 62–63
in thoracentesis, *100*
Loculated pleural fluid
in radiographic findings, 26
in ultrasonographic findings, 40f, *42*
Lorazepam, 66
Louis, angle of, 3
Lung abscess
versus bronchopleural fistula, 30, *34*
radiographic findings, 30
Lung biopsy, open versus thoracoscopic, *173*
Lung puncture, closed-tube thoracostomy and, 135
Lungs
anatomy, 6–7
physical examination, 13–20
physiology and pleuropulmonary relationships, 7–8
in pleural cavity, 7
Lymphatics, anatomy, 6
Lymphocytosis, pleural fluid, 80
Lymphoid cells, pleural, 8

M
Magnetic resonance imaging, 22
Malignant mesothelioma, *33,* 84
closed-needle pleural biopsy and, *112*
Marcaine (bupivacaine), 64
Meclofenamate, 69
Meclomen (meclofenamate), 69
Medical notes. *See* Documentation
Menghini biopsy needle, 116f–117f, 117–118
Meperidine, 71
for pain alleviation in pleurodesis, 158
Mepivacaine, 64
Mesothelial cells, in pleural fluid, 80, *85*
Mesothelioma, malignant. *See* Malignant mesothelioma
Metastatic pleural disease, treatment problems, *76*
Midazolam, 66
Minocycline, 156
Mitoxantrone, 156
Morphine sulfate, 70
continuous intravenous infusion, 70
immediate- and sustained-release preparations, 71
intramuscular administration, 70–71
oral preparations, 71
Motrin (ibuprofen), 69
MRI (magnetic resonance imaging), 22
Multiple-pass coaxial system needles, for fine-needle aspiration biopsy, 118
versus single-pass systems, *125*

Mupirocin, topical application, 62
Muscles
  anterolateral chest, 4, 4f
  intercostal, 5
  posterolateral chest, 4, 5f
  for respiration control, *10*

N

Naloxone hydrochloride, 72
Naprosyn (naproxen), 69
Naproxen, 69
Narcan (naloxone hydrochloride), 72
Nausea, as opioid adverse effect, 72
Needles
  for fine-needle aspiration biopsy, 116–118, 116f–117f
  for pleural biopsy, 105–106, 106f–108f, 108
    safe use, *112*
  for thoracocentesis, 93, 94f
    technique, 96–98
Neomycin, topical application, 62
Nerves, intercostal, 6
Neuropathic pain, *76*
Nociceptive pain, *76*
Nodules, pleural, 28, 28f
  fine-needle aspiration biopsy, 121f, 124
Nonsteroidal antiinflammatory drugs, 69
  adverse reactions to, 69
  commonly used, 69–70
Nortriptyline, 74
Notes. *See* Documentation
Novocaine (procaine hydrochloride), 64–65
NSAIDs. *See* Nonsteroidal antiinflammatory drugs

O

Oblique views, of chest, 21
Ointments, antimicrobial. *See* Topical antimicrobial ointments
Open lung biopsy, thoracoscopic lung biopsy versus, *173*
Opioids, 70–72. *See also* Morphine; *specific opioid*
  adverse effects, 72–73
Oxycodone, 71

P

Pain
  analgesia for. *See* Analgesics
  defined, 67
  nociceptive versus neuropathic, *76*
  in pleural disease, 13
  in pleurodesis
    alleviation, 158
    prevention, *160*
  from thoracoscopy, *74,* 170
Pain syndromes, after thoracoscopy and thoracotomy, 74
Palpation
  anatomic landmarks for, 16
  in pleural effusions, 18
  in pneumothorax, 18
Paracetic acid sterilization, 58
Paramalignant pleural effusions, 84
  chest tube placement and, *85, 88*
Parapneumonic effusions, complicated, 81–82
Parenchymal disease, pleural abnormalities versus, 30–31, 31f
Parham bands, 146, *150*
Parietal pleura, 6
  biopsies, thoracoscopy for, 167–168, 169f
Patient-controlled analgesia, *76*
Patient history, prior to thoracoscopy, 172–173
Patient record. *See* Documentation
PCA (patient-controlled analgesia), *76*
PCNA (percutaneous needle aspiration). *See* Fine-needle aspiration biopsy
Percocet (oxycodone), 71
Percodan (oxycodone), 71
Percussion
  indirect technique, 19
  in physical examination, 16
  in pleural effusions, 18
  in pneumothorax, 18
Percutaneous needle aspiration. *See* Fine-needle aspiration biopsy
pH, pleural fluid, 80, *85*
Phenylbutazone, 70
pHisohex (hexachlorophene), 55
Phrenic nerve, in thoracic cage anatomy, 3
Physical dependence, on opioids, 72, 74
Physical examination, in pleural disease, 13–17
  clinical recommendations, 18–19
  pleural effusion, 17–18
  pneumothorax, 18
  prior to thoracoscopy, 172–173
Piroxicam, 70
Pleura
  physical examination, 13–20
  physiology and fluid movement in, 8–9
  and pleuropulmonary relationships, 7–8
  radiologic examination, 21–35. *See also* Pleural radiology

ultrasonographic examination, 37–43. *See also* Ultrasonography
visceral versus parietal, 6–7
Pleural cavity, anatomy, 6–7
Pleural disease. *See also specific conditions*
differential diagnosis, 79–88
metastatic, treatment problems, *76*
multidisciplinary team approach to, 79
pharmacologic agents used in, 61–76
analgesics, 67–73
antidepressants, 73–74
anxiolytics, hypnotics, and sedatives, 65–67
local anesthetics, 62–65
topical antimicrobial ointments, 61–62
physical examination in, 13–17
clinical recommendations, 18–19
pleural effusion, 17–18
pneumothorax, 18
prior to thoracoscopy, 172–173
signs and symptoms
major, 13
miscellaneous, 19
Pleural effusions, 8
atypical appearance, *33*
chylothorax and, 84
diagnosis, 79
differential diagnosis, 79–81, 86t–87t
empyema and. *See* Empyema
hemothorax and. *See* Hemothorax
malignant, pleurodesis for, *88*
management, 81–82, 85
paramalignant, 84, *85, 88*
parapneumonic, 81–82
physical findings in, 17–18
from postcardiac injury syndrome, 84–85
pulmonary embolism/infarction causing, 85
pulmonary function tests in, *19–20*
radiographic findings, 26–27, 27f
free-flowing, 26
large, 26
loculations and, 26
small (subpulmonic), 26–27
ultrasonographic findings, 41f
Pleural fibrosis. *See* Fibrosis, pleural; Fibrothorax
Pleural fluid
absence of, closed-needle pleural biopsy and, *112*
and air-fluid level, 29–30, 30f
appearance and components, 80
free-flowing versus loculated
radiographic findings, 26
ultrasonographic findings, *39f–40f, 42*
lateral decubitus film for, *34*
mesothelial cells in, 80, *85*
movement, 8–9
pH of, 80, *85*
in pleural effusion differential diagnosis, 79–80
in pleural radiology, 24–25, 32
from thoracentesis, 98, 99
Pleural nodules. *See* Nodules, pleural
Pleural plaques, visualization, *34*
Pleural pressure
defined, 8
gradient, 8
Pleural procedures. *See individual procedures*
Pleural radiology, 21–35
abnormal findings
lung abscess and empyema, 30
versus parenchymal or extrapleural disease, 30–31, 31f
parietal and visceral, describing, 24–26
pleural effusions, 26–27, 27f
pleural thickening and fibrosis, 27–28, 28f
pneumothorax, 29–30, 29f–30f
clinical recommendations, 32–33
complications, 31–32
contraindications, 22–23
defined, 21
equipment and techniques, 23–31
indications, 22
normal pleural anatomy on, 23–24, 24f
principles, 21–22
Pleural reflections, in pleural radiology, 23
Pleural thickening
diagnosis, 83
management, 83
pulmonary function tests in, *19–20*
radiographic findings, 27–28, 28f
Pleur-Evac chest drainage system, 47, 48f
Pleurodesis, 155–161
agents used for, 155–156
variability of results and, *159*
complications, 158
contraindications, 155
defined, 155
documentation requirements, 158
equipment, 155–156
indications, 155
for pleural effusions, 81
malignant, *88*

Pleurodesis *(cont'd)*
for pneumothorax, 83
procedural guidelines, 160
rotation after, *160*
techniques, 156–158, 157f
Pneumothorax
catamenial, *88*
diagnosis, 83
management, 83
open, *149*
physical findings in, 18
radiographic findings, 29–30, 29f–30f
secondary, 83
spontaneous, 83
tension physiology and, 32–33
thoracentesis and, 99
Polymyxin B, topical application, 62
Pontocaine (tetracaine), 65
Pores of Wang, 8
Posterior intercostal arteries, 5
Povidone-iodine, 55
Procaine hydrochloride, 64–65
Procedures. *See individual procedures*
Prophylaxis
endocarditis, *75*
prior to thoracoscopy, *75*
Pseudochylous effusions, 81
Psychological dependence, on opioids, 72–73, 74
Pulmonary edema, reexpansion, thoracentesis and, 99
Pulmonary function tests, indications for, *19*
Pulmonary ligaments, in pleural radiology, 23–24

R
Radiology, pleural. *See* Pleural radiology
"Reach tulip" mnemonic, 80
Record-keeping. *See* Documentation
Recumbent views, of chest, 21
Reexpansion pulmonary edema, thoracentesis and, 99, *100*
Respiration, muscles controlling, *10*
Respiratory depression
after drug administration, 74
opioids causing, 72
Right lung, 7
Romazicon (flumazenil), 66–67
Rounded atelectasis, *33–34*

S
Sclerosing agents, in pleurodesis, 155–156
Secondary pneumothorax, 83
Sedatives, 65–67
agents used as, 66–67. *See also* Anxiolytics
Seldinger technique, 130, 131f, 132
Serterner, Friedrich Wilhelm, 74
Skin degerming, 53–59. *See also* Disinfection
agents used for, 55–56
labeling information, 58
washing off, 58
complications, 58
defined, 53
handwashing and, 58
indications, 55
procedures for, 54
techniques, 55
Skin folds, in pleural radiology, 32
Small-bore chest tubes, for closed-tube thoracostomy. *See under* Closed-tube thoracostomy
Sound waves, described, 37, 37f
Spontaneous pneumothorax, 83
Starling's law of transcapillary exchange, 8–9
Steam sterilization, 57
Sterile packaging, expiration dates on, *59*
Sterilization, 53–59
complications, 58
defined, 53
indications, 55
procedures for, 54–55
techniques, 57–58
Stomas, pleural, 8
Subpulmonic pleural effusions, 26–27, 27f
Suction pumps, portable, 45
Surgical scrub
agents used for, 55–56
preparation for, *59*
prior to thoracoscopy, *59*
Surveillance notes, chest drainage device, 21

T
Talc pleurodesis, 156, 157, 157f
for pleural effusion, 81
Talc slurry
cancer and, *159*
described, *159*
for pleurodesis, 156
Tension physiology, pneumothorax and, 32–33
Tetracaine, 65
Tetracycline, pleurodesis and, *159*
Tetracycline derivatives, 156
Thal-Quick chest tube set, 140, 141f
Thoracentesis, 93–102
anatomical landmarks for, *9*
avoiding intercostal vessels in, *10*

complications, 99
contraindications, 93
defined, 93
documentation requirements, 98–99
equipment, 93
exploratory, prior to closed-tube thoracostomy, 134, 140
indications, 93
patient position for, 94, 95f
procedural guidelines, *101*
techniques, 93–99
using ultrasonographic guidance, 38–40
Thoracic cage, anatomy, 3–4, 4f–5f
Thoracic drainage devices
collection chamber in, 45
complications, 49–50
contraindications, 46
current versus old systems, *50*
defined, 45
documentation requirements, 49
"dry" versus "wet" suction devices, 52
equipment, 46–47, 47f–48f
fluid measurement and, *51*
follow-up chest radiograph, 49
indications, 46
leaks in, *51*
principles, 45
suction control chamber in, 45, 50
techniques and setting-up, 48–49
water seal chamber, 45
air leaks in, 50
versus negative suction, *51*
and tube disconnection, *51–52*
Thoracoscopic lung biopsy, open lung biopsy versus, *173*
Thoracoscopy, 163–174
complications, 171–172
avoiding, *173*
contraindications, 163–164
defined, 163
documentation requirements, 170–171
equipment, 164–165, 164f–165f
follow-up observations, *173–174*
indications, 163
for lung biopsy, open lung biopsy versus, *173*
pain syndromes after, 74
patient position for, 166–167, 166f
in pleural effusion, 81
procedural guidelines, 174
prophylactic antibiotics prior to, *75*
techniques, 165–171, 166f, 168f–170f, 173
Thoracostomy, closed-tube. *See* Closed-tube thoracostomy
Thoracotomy, pain syndromes after, 74
Thora-Seal III chest drainage system, 47–48, 48f
Three-container system, thoracic drainage device, 45
Tolerance, to analgesics, 68
Topical antimicrobial ointments, 61–62
adverse effects, 62
agents used in, 62
for chest tube wounds, *75*
contraindications, 61
indications, 61
principles of use, 61
Toradol (ketorolac), 70
Trachea, in pleural cavity anatomy, 7
Transcapillary exchange, Starling's law of, 8–9
Transthoracic needle aspiration. *See* Fine-needle aspiration biopsy
Transthoracic needle biopsy. *See* Fine-needle aspiration biopsy
Transudate
defined, *10*
in pleural effusion differential diagnosis, 79
"Trapped lung," *88*
Triglyceride levels, in pleural fluid, 81
Tru-close thoracic vent, 127
TTNA (transthoracic needle aspiration). *See* Fine-needle aspiration biopsy
TTNB (transthoracic needle biopsy). *See* Fine-needle aspiration biopsy
Tubes. *See* Chest tubes
Turner biopsy needle, for fine-needle aspiration biopsy, 116, 116f–117f
Two percent glutaraldehyde, 57
Tylenol. *See* Acetaminophen

U

Ultrasonography
advantages, *42*
complications, 41
contraindications, 38
defined, 37
documentation requirements, 40
equipment, 38
frequency and imaging depth, 37, 37f, 41
gray scale sections, 38, 42
indications, 38
interpretation of images, 42
principles, 37–38, 37f
technique, 38–40, 39f–41f
timing, 41–42

V

Valium (diazepam), 66
Van Sonnenberg sump catheters, 103, 128, 130f
Vasoconstrictors, use with local anesthetics, 63
Vasovagal reactions, thoracentesis and, 99
VATS (video-assisted thoracoscopic surgery), 163, 170f
Veins, intercostal, 6
Versed (midazolam), 66
Vicodin (hydrocodone), 71
Video-assisted thoracoscopic surgery, 163, 170f
Visceral pleura, 6
Vistaril (hydroxyzine), 67
Voltaren (diclofenac), 69

W

Wang, pores of, 8
Wavelength, ultrasonographic, 37, 37f
"White-out," hemithorax, 26
Wounds, chest tube
  dehiscence at incision site, *75–76*
  dressings for, after closed-tube thoracostomy, 145–146, 147f
  perioperative infection
    prevention, *75*
    risk, *74–75*
  topical antiseptic ointments for, *75*

X

Xylocaine (lidocaine hydrochloride), 64